**Praise for *Be***

*"This book is very timely! It is a book that all professionals would want to purchase. It addresses professional humility and goes far beyond medicine.*

*Knowing that doctors have the responsibility of saving lives, it is also good to realize that getting to know their patients is of equal importance for the good of the patient and of the physician.*

*Much is dependent on the attitude of the doctor when it comes to relating to and properly understanding the individual that they are treating. As we are aware, we are fortunate in The Bahamas to have medical professionals, including doctors, who have excelled in various fields.*

*This book can help to serve as a valuable resource to further enhance their ability to better relate to their patients and to others."*

**– Her Excellency, The Most Honorable Dame Cynthia (Mother) A. Pratt**, ON, GCMG, GB, CD, JP Governor General of The Commonwealth of The Bahamas

*"Dr. Parker's maiden effort is a keeper. Her thorough grasp of the art and science of medicine; combined with her personable and intimate style, makes this a captivating, enjoyable read. This should be a fixture on the reading list of every physician...everywhere! Bravo!"*

– **Dr. Duane E. Sands**, M.D., F.A.C.S., Former Minister of Health, Commonwealth of The Bahamas (2017–2020)

*"Dr. Kristine Parker-Curling has done an outstanding job with Beyond the Knowledge, offering a deeply personal and compelling exploration of her experiences in medicine. Her willingness to bear her soul and share numerous personal stories make this book both powerful and relatable. What sets this book apart is its authenticity – Dr. Parker does not shy away from the challenges, emotions, and ethical dilemmas that come with practicing medicine. Her stories resonate deeply, and many readers will recognize parallels in their own journeys. This should, and I predict will, be a recommended resource for medical students and young physicians that will hopefully help to influence positive changes in behaviour and shape a more empathetic and self-aware generation of doctors."*

– **Dr. Corrine Sin Quee**, Director, UWI School of Clinical Medicine and Research, The Bahamas

*"Beyond the Knowledge is an indispensable compendium for every physician, illuminating key steps to elevate our practice of healthcare delivery through compassion, awareness, responsiveness, and engagement. Dr. Kristine Parker-Curling has provided a captivating read that is not only transformative but also empowering us to connect deeply with our patients. I urge all physicians, those emerging and seasoned, to embrace this invaluable resource, as it fills a perceived void in our training and inspires us to practice medicine with a genuine human touch. Thank you, Dr. Parker-Curling, for this essential blueprint and vital contribution!"*

– **Dr. Gemma Annwen Rolle**, President of the Medical Association of The Bahamas

*"Beyond the Knowledge: Power Steps for Compassionate Care is a wonderful guide to the often-overlooked human side of medicine. As an endocrinologist and obesity medicine specialist physician trained in multiple social settings (Jamaica, Bahamas & USA) she has a unique perspective about building trust, breaking bad news with compassion, and maintaining empathy amid burnout. Her RACE/C.A.R.E. framework offers a roadmap for transforming day to day clinical interactions into meaningful connections. It's a proud moment for me as a teacher to see Dr. Kristine Parker-Curling transform the lessons we once shared into a groundbreaking guide for patient-centered care. Her book not only reflects the foundational ideas that we discussed but elevates them with her unique vision and compassion. The student has truly become the teacher, setting a new standard for empathy and innovation in medicine."*

– **Dr. Srikanth Garikaparthi**, Consultant Plastic Surgeon & Lecturer, Surgery; School of Clinical Medicine & Research; University of West Indies

*"This book is a powerful guide for healthcare professionals, focusing on compassion, awareness, responsiveness, and engagement. It highlights the importance of communication, trust, and professionalism in patient care. The sections on listening, eye contact, and adapting communication are especially insightful. It also addresses modern challenges like telemedicine and AI in healthcare.*
*This book is a must-read for medical professionals seeking to enhance their patient interactions."*

– **Soonho Kwon, M.D., M.S.**; Professor of Medicine; Director of Thyroid Procedure Clinic; Division of Endocrinology; Department of Internal Medicine; Medical University of South Carolina

*"Beyond The Knowledge: Power Steps For Doctoring With A Human Touch is a valuable resource for health professionals looking to enhance their communication skills and improve patient experiences. The author emphasizes the importance of incorporating compassion, empathy, and self-awareness into medical practice.*

*We should all strive to provide holistic patient care by acknowledging and addressing the emotional and psychological aspects of a patient's well-being. The book would be a useful guide for professionals at any stage of their careers, providing them with practical steps to engage with patients more meaningfully. The emphasis on creating an environment of trust and compassion is a key takeaway, as this is what truly elevates patient care."*

– **Jyotika K Fernandes, MD**; Wendy and Keith Wellin Endowed Chair in Endocrinology; Professor of Medicine; Division of Endocrinology, Diabetes & Metabolic Diseases; Department of Medicine; Medical University of South Carolina; Endocrine Section Chief, RHJ VA Medical Centre, Charleston SC

*"Dr. Kristine, congratulations on this incredible book which I consider a breath of fresh air. With more than 30 years serving seniors, this should be required reading for practitioners. Beyond The Knowledge permits us to imagine a physician who combines compassion and empathy, making patients feel heard and valued through attentive listening, eye contact, and a reassuring touch. These soft skills create an environment of trust that can make or break the patient experience. While exceptional diagnostic skills are important, possessing these soft skills fosters trust and confidence.*

*Practitioners who are approachable and warm, create a safe environment where patients feel comfortable discussing their concerns, leading to better health outcomes. Bravo to you on an exceptional piece!"*

– **Jeremy Neely,** MBA, NHA, CASP

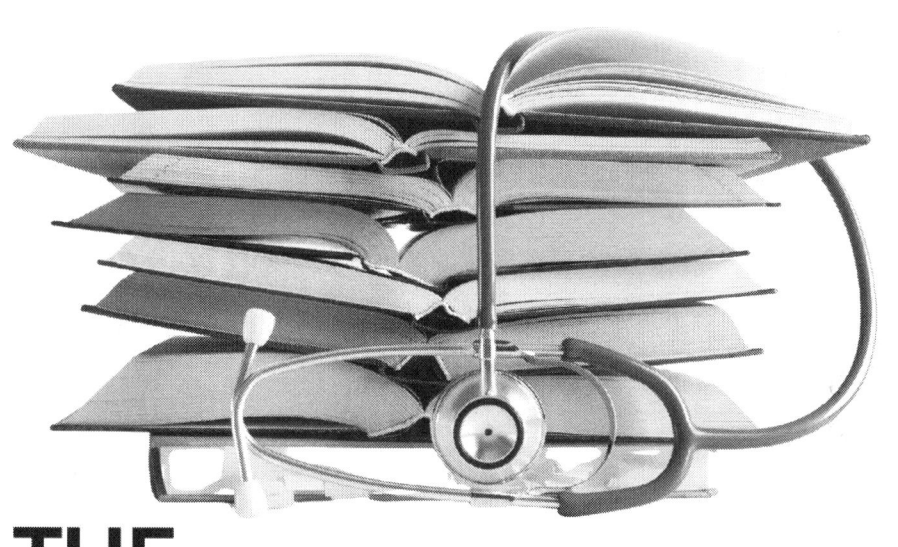

# BEYOND
## THE
## KNOWLEDGE

# BEYOND THE KNOWLEDGE

*Power Steps For Doctoring With A Human Touch*

## DR. KRISTINE PARKER-CURLING

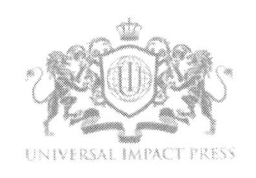

UNIVERSAL IMPACT PRESS

Copyright © 2024 by Dr. Krisitne Parker-Curling. All rights reserved.

Published by Universal Impact Press, an Imprint of Arete Media International. www.AreteMediaInternational.com

No part of this publication may be reproduced, distributed, or transmitted in any form or by any means, including photocopying, recording, or other electronic or mechanical methods, without the prior written permission of the publisher, except in the case of brief quotations embodied in critical reviews and certain other noncommercial uses permitted by copyright law. For permission requests, please contact the publisher.

The content of this book, including text, images, graphics, and the cover design, is copyrighted by Dr. Kristine Parker-Curling. Certain images and graphics were created by Universal Impact Press and are used with permission.

All referenced Scripture has been taken from the Holy Bible, New International Version®, NIV®. Copyright © 1973, 1978, 1984, 2011 by Biblica, Inc.™ Used by permission of Zondervan. All rights reserved worldwide. www.zondervan.com. The NIV and New International Version are trademarks registered in the United States Patent and Trademark Office by Biblica, Inc.™

This book is intended to provide general information and insights about the practice of medicine and the doctor-patient relationship. The author and publisher have used their best efforts in preparing this book and the information provided herein is for educational purposes only. The information, advice, and strategies contained herein may not be suitable for every situation. The author and publisher are not herein engaged in rendering professional services, and the reader should consult with a professional where appropriate. Neither the publisher nor the author shall be liable for any loss of profit or any other commercial damages, including but not limited to special, incidental, consequential, or other damages.

The patient stories and anecdotes shared in this book are based on the author's imagination and experiences and have been modified to protect patient privacy and confidentiality. Any resemblance to actual persons, living or dead, or actual events is purely coincidental. For personal effect, common colors are periodically used for surnames of patients or physicians in this writing. This book may contain links to external websites. These links are provided as a convenience and for informational purposes only. The author and publisher bear no responsibility for the accuracy, legality, or content of the external site or for that of subsequent links.

Paperback ISBN: 978-1-956711-79-0; Hardcover ISBN: 978-1-956711-80-6

# Dedication

I have been fortunate enough in life to encounter many people who have had the opportunity to positively influence me.

I wish to thank those who are still in the land of the living.

To my immediate family still here to share with me: Mom, my siblings, my husband, and my children, I love you. You have been a dedicated family and support system!

To my mentors, it truly takes a village!

This work is dedicated to those people with whom I have had the chance to directly interact, who continue to influence me even though they have transitioned to a higher calling.

To my dad, who never got to see my finished product but who, in his weakness, read enough to encourage me to keep going and to reassure me that my book was 'worth being written.' I love you, Dad.

To Grampy, who told me that the meaning of life was to make my life so meaningful that even when I am gone, someone would desire to imitate me.

To my nephew, shine on.

To my cousins who have gone on before us: we shared so many memories and grew up together as siblings do. You live on in all of us, and we remember you fondly and miss you dearly.

To my aunts and uncles who have journeyed on before us, you influenced us in so many ways, and we are forever grateful.

# Contents

| | |
|---|---|
| Inspiration For This Book | 1 |
| Preface | 3 |
| Introduction | 7 |
| SECTION 1: COMPASSION | 17 |
| 1. The Power of Compassion | 21 |
| The Power of Compassion<br>Part 2: Cultivating Compassion Among Colleagues | 31 |
| The Power of Compassion<br>Part 3: Self-Compassion: The Foundation of Caregiving | 41 |
| 2. The Power of Acknowledgement | 55 |
| 3. The Power of Courtesy | 63 |
| SECTION 2: AWARENESS | 75 |
| 4. The Power of Your Physical Positioning in the Room | 79 |
| 5. The Power of Listening | 85 |
| The Power of Listening<br>Part 2: The Diagnostic Value of Listening | 93 |

| | |
|---|---|
| The Power of Listening | 101 |
| Part 3: Listening Beyond the Obvious | |
| 6. The Power of Eye Contact | 109 |
| SECTION 3: REPONSIVENESS | 117 |
| 7. The Power of Touch | 121 |
| 8. The Power of Effective Communication | 131 |
| The Power of Effective Communication | 139 |
| Part 2: Adapting Communication to Patient Needs | |
| The Power Effective Communication | 145 |
| Part 3: Communication in Sensitive Scenarios | |
| 9. The Power of Trust | 153 |
| 10. The Power of Referring | 161 |
| 11. The Power of Professionalism In Your Office | 169 |
| SECTION 4: ENGAGEMENT | 175 |
| 12. The Power of Relatability | 179 |
| 13. The Power of Navigating Difficult Patient Scenarios Well | 195 |
| The Power of Navigating Difficult Patient Scenarios Well | 201 |
| Part 2: Breaking Bad News | |
| The Power of Navigating Difficult Patient Scenarios Well | 209 |
| Part 3: Talking About Sex | |

| | |
|---|---|
| The Power of Navigating Difficult Patient Scenarios Well | 217 |

Part 4: Fertility Issues

| | | |
|---|---|---|
| 14. | The Power of Serving as The Doctor to A Doctor | 227 |
| 15. | The Power of Caring for the Patient Whose Close Family Member is A Physician | 239 |
| 16. | The Power of Doctoring in The Age of Telemedicine | 247 |
| 17. | The Power of Doctoring in The Age of Artificial Intelligence | 257 |

| | |
|---|---|
| Epilogue | 265 |
| Afterword | 267 |
| Acknowledgments | 269 |
| Bonus Resources | 271 |
| Power Steps | 273 |
| C.A.R.E. Quick Reference Guide | 275 |
| Self Care Essentials | 276 |
| C.A.R.E. Self-Assessment | 277 |
| Prayers for Physicians | 279 |
| Endnotes | 281 |
| Meet Dr. Kristine | 285 |
| Index | 287 |

# Inspiration For This Book

In early 2023, I joined a course alongside seven other wonderful 'classmates' to learn how to share 'our stories'. We had the unique opportunity to engage with a legendary motivational speaker and receive personal feedback.

During that course, my perspective on life shifted significantly. I was encouraged to use my experiences to inspire others, with the insight that the personal development space could be where I thrive. My journey, marked by overcoming challenges, positioned me well to make a meaningful impact in this field.

I realized I had a compelling story to tell. Along with my classmates, I was motivated to start sharing it. The course was both enlightening and freeing, allowing me to connect deeply with the experiences of others and find joy in their revelations, both public and private. By the end of it, I was inspired to start writing this book, beginning my work on the very night the course concluded.

I had always sensed I was meant to write, yet the idea of starting something significant felt daunting. Unsure of my first project's direction, what I began writing that night deviated entirely from my expectations. However, as I typed, the concept and structure of the book unfolded naturally. I had found my flow, leading to the creation of the 'Beyond The Knowledge' series. To date, I've written three children's books, inspired by my children, but this book felt urgent, a project I needed to complete.

Following the course, a meeting filled with encouragement and challenge solidified my belief in the importance of my writing in this niche. With my husband's encouragement and support, I continued to write amidst a busy life. Even after long days, I found the strength to write, sometimes managing only a few paragraphs.

The rest, as they say, is history.

# Preface

Professional and personal development are inherent in the practice of medicine and generally mandatory in most settings. Typically, to maintain a medical license to practice, a physician must participate in some form of 'continuing medical education,' which serves to keep them updated and abreast of new standards of practice in the ever-changing field of medicine.

As medical knowledge evolves, with new discoveries made, knowledge becomes outdated and updated relatively quickly. A 10-year period could see an entire paradigm shift in some fields of medicine as new information renders what we previously knew obsolete.

This need for continued updating and knowledge acquisition is not upsetting to me; in fact, I find excitement in attending conferences and paying attention to lectures.

I am one of those individuals who feels they are missing out if I attend one lecture when there is a choice of multiple topics running simultaneously on the schedule. It's quite frustrating having multiple lectures running at the same time because, how are we expected to attend all the lectures if there are competing topics being presented simultaneously?

Yes, I'm that person at the plenary at 8 AM, seated somewhere in the first few rows. I just can't help it! Don't judge me. I feel guilty if I miss it, lol.

## *The Gap in Medical Education*

From the time one contemplates medical school, to the time one becomes a physician, generalist, specialist, or subspecialist, one is engaged in continuous learning activities. Throughout the years of the practice of medicine and the training for the practice of medicine, there is a paucity of time that I can recall being taught how to interact with a patient.

We learned how to 'take a history' (gather relevant information about the patient), 'perform a physical exam,' and present the 'case' to the resident (the more senior of the 'junior doctors'), the team, and the attending physician (consultant or boss/head doctor).

We learned how to read the results of lab tests and how to interpret many common results. We know how to interpret basic radiographs and to read imaging reports and relate them to the clinical presentation of 'the case' to formulate the plan.

## *Learning Through Experience*

I had many experiences during my training and practice that taught me how not to interact with patients because if you paid enough attention to their reactions, you could see which actions were well received and which were not at all well received.

However, I never had any formal training or even discussion that could guide me on how to navigate the actual effective communication with my patients.

We hear of good 'bedside manner,' but what is that anyway? And who was supposed to teach that to me? Did I somehow miss that class? Does anyone even care about that?

I suppose there was some implicit learning because we obviously had to observe our seniors and 'teachers' or attendings or consultants interacting with patients and staff; but what you would see would be very dependent on who you were learning from, their personality, their mood, the practice setting, their specialty, and many other variables that you would not have been astute enough to dissect and interpret appropriately.

And admittedly, not everything that we observed and did would be considered desirable behavior.

## *The Knack for Patient Interaction*

I did discover eventually that I have a 'knack' for interacting with patients and this was really luck of the draw. I got dealt the personality card and did not even know it. Quite frankly, it would be the patient's reactions to me or their overt words to me that would positively reinforce certain behaviors that may have come naturally to me and not to others.

This is not to say that others aren't excellent and skilled physicians or that they are not providing excellent care for their patients, but it caused me to wonder if there was a particular skill set that caused one physician to stand out in their relatability and or likeability to patients.

The next question was, can this skill be identified, expanded on, and taught, and finally, the question became, were these identifiable qualities of a physician with 'excellent bedside manner' described in any formal way?

Even if there was not one composite or comprehensive writing on the matter, were there studies or writings that could help to substantiate these qualities that I identified and described as being useful and effective tools for enhancing the physician-patient relationship?

As I wrote this book and did the research to substantiate what I described as the characteristics or actions that caused patients to respond positively to myself and to certain other physicians, I did find evidence to support these statements.

## *The Aim of This Book*

The aim of this project was to compile a concise handbook, so to speak, of skills that a physician, nurse, nurse practitioner, physician assistant, physical therapist, or any caregiver can develop to improve his or her ability to relate effectively to patients, and people in general.

As we race through the tasks that need completion, sometimes we need to be reminded to care, not only for others but for ourselves also. In addition to improving patient communication, we need to remind ourselves that maintaining balance in our own lives is of paramount importance and will help to enhance our professional longevity.

We have so much to read already, so brevity was a priority while trying not to sacrifice detail. Of course, the degree to which you implement each of these tools will depend on your specialty, gender, age, your patient population, practice setting, your personality, your existing skillset, and your comfort level. You don't want your interactions to appear contrived.

Of course, a radiologist or a pathologist may need to focus on a different skill set than a pediatrician would. A trauma surgeon and a gynecologist probably would have different needs when it comes to skill development in this regard.

So, here's to a brief review of some of the things that they didn't formally teach us in medical (or other professional) training that might go a long way toward making you more well-rounded as a physician and caregiver.

We can all pass tests, we have proven that on many occasions, now let's learn to talk to patients and delve 'BEYOND THE KNOWLEDGE'!

*Dr. Kristine Parker-Curling*

# Introduction

Professionally, I am an Endocrinologist, Internist, and Obesity Medicine Specialist, as well as a public speaker, associate lecturer, and author (now published). My journey through undergraduate studies, medical school, residency, fellowship, and into my medical practice continually revealed my innate abilities in relating to people, including my patients.

Undoubtedly, I am a born communicator, coming from a family of communicators. My undergraduate studies in psychology further reinforced my skills in interpersonal communication.

I graduated *Summa Cum Laude* with a double major in Biology and Psychology before matriculating into medical school, where I graduated with many awards, including 'most outstanding student' or valedictorian. I continue to explore and develop professionally and personally.

## *The Genesis of a Communication Tool*

Given my lack of formal training in the areas of 'relating to' and 'communicating with' patients, I set out to develop a tool that could serve as a resource for medical students, residents, fellows, practicing physicians, physician organizations, and other healthcare professionals in mastering the art of relationship building.

The principles discussed in this book can serve as practical guidelines for communicating with colleagues and other staff in the hospital, healthcare settings, and indeed any work or professional setting. Effective and empathetic communication can endear people to you, motivating them to perform tasks for you that are far above and beyond their call of duty.

This tool is crucial, regardless of the sphere of communication in which you function.

## *Empathy in Action*

Asking someone to do something is so much more effective and pleasant than telling someone to do it, even if it is their job to do it!

It's the little things that cause the unit clerk to bring you coffee when she goes on her break to get her own. It's the little things that prompt the nurse to look out for you and not wake you up unless it's truly necessary (yes, you can catch a teeny tiny nap while on call overnight or on night float if you really need it). It's the little things that can influence whether you get that fellowship spot or not.

You passed several team members before you got to the program director's office for the interview. Did you say good morning to the staff members, or did you glide through the corridor wearing your 'doctor cape' and 'crown of condescension and arrogance'? Think about it!

Sure, you were the smartest resident, sure you were the chief resident, and you probably got the highest score on the board exam...but do people like you? Do they want to work with you? Or do they want to get their work done as quickly as possible to avoid interacting with you?

The 'staff members' you so flippantly bypassed may have more to do with the decision-making process than you can imagine. They have seen many of us come and go, and they have a pretty good inclination about who will fit in with their program and who most certainly will not! So be aware and remember that everyone you encounter plays a role.

## *Communication: A Learnable Skill*

The ability to communicate well, though so obviously necessary, is not innate and does not come naturally to some people. This is surprisingly true with doctors, in my experience.

The great news is that effective communication is indeed a skill, and becoming an excellent and confident communicator is within your reach! You CAN learn to communicate well and to communicate effectively with those around you, especially your patients!

As you journey through this book, you will start to unlock some of the power to communicate that you didn't even realize you had.

Through stories that you can most certainly relate to in many cases, you will be given the opportunity to reflect on how you would have responded in similar scenarios, or how you responded in the exact same scenario. You can think about how you would have handled it, how I handled it, how the doctor described handled it, and what could have been done differently.

You will start to consider the patient's reaction to you, your words, your body language, and other nonverbal cues that you may be giving off. You may even begin to see why people respond to you the way that they do, positively or otherwise.

At the end of this experience, you will emerge a more confident communicator, and you can immediately, even while reading the book, start to implement some of the principles that you will learn, and you will see them affect your day-to-day interactions almost immediately. If there were a class on empathetic, effective, and efficient communication, this is it!

## *The Importance of Self-Communication*

In learning how to communicate with others, it is so important that we also learn to communicate with ourselves. We must learn to listen to our bodies and become more attuned to our own physical, emotional, spiritual, and mental health. What is happening inside us as humans will influence what we give off as caregivers.

As much as we try to compartmentalize our lives, it is impossible to truly divorce ourselves from our feelings, emotions, experiences, opinions, symptoms, and all other aspects of ourselves. This is why coming to grips with our humanity, in all its uniqueness, allows us to take our caregiving to another level.

When we address and feed our own needs and become more whole as people, we can become more effective as doctors and this allows for a more meaningful connection with our patients and with others.

After all, the thing that separates us from machines is indeed our humanity.

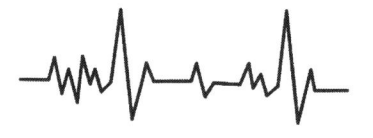

## The RACE and C.A.R.E Framework

In this writing, we will explore doctoring within the RACE and C.A.R.E. framework.

This RACE/C.A.R.E. framework will address the need for compassion, awareness, responsiveness, and engagement in our interactions and can serve as a reminder for us as we interact with people on a day-to-day basis.

We will take a deep dive into each one of these themes so that we can enhance our skills and truly become doctors that C.A.R.E.

## *Integrating Essential Skills in Medical Education*

So, let's integrate these important skills into our formal training as medical students, residents, fellows, nursing students, pharmacy students, PA students, PT students, and allied health professionals.

Let's include these most important messages in our CME's as practicing physicians and professionals.

Let's reinforce it during the 'onboarding' of new staff members at our integrated healthcare systems and hospitals. Let us go 'BEYOND THE KNOWLEDGE'!

**As you RACE through your day, don't forget to C.A.R.E.**

## *The Value of Acronyms in Learning*

We have spent most of our academic lives learning and utilizing acronyms. These are very familiar learning and memory tools.

There are still a few of them that I remember and use with regularity, and many find them extremely helpful if only to help organize initial understanding.

When we think about the importance of our relationships then we can recognize the necessity for great communication and self-care.

The RACE and C.A.R.E. framework will help us to organize ourselves as we navigate and perfect the power steps on doctoring with a human touch.

As physicians that C.A.R.E. we all recognize the need to build our capacity for the qualities outlined by this framework and will explore how we can examine our situations and make changes to improve ourselves.

## *Applying the Framework in Various Settings*

The power steps that we will navigate will be organized into sections based on the RACE and C.A.R.E framework which can help the practitioner who is working in a long-term healthcare facility, or one who has to 'RACE' through a busy clinic.

**Just remember that RACE rearranged, spells C.A.R.E**, and you can apply these tenants to any scenario. You will likely find that the RACE/C.A.R.E. framework applies to the effective management of other interpersonal relationships that you will have to navigate. Let's break it down just a little bit.

## *Deep Dive into the Components of C.A.R.E*

The 'C' in C.A.R.E. stands for '**COMPASSION**' and in these chapters, we will be reminded of the need to be compassionate in our approaches to patients, colleagues, and ourselves.

We will discuss and master several power steps in this chapter that will help us to improve and perfect our ability to practice compassionately, while still leaving some room for ourselves.

The 'A' stands for **'AWARENESS'** and speaks to the need to be aware of yourself and what you bring to the encounter. We will also learn to pay attention to what is happening with others in the room. This can provide valuable information that can enhance our ability to gain more than what is spoken from the encounter.

We will be reminded to pay attention to the needs of the patient and of those with whom we interact. One can be present and not attentive to the goings on around them and the power steps explored in this section will highlight some of the major factors that require our attention in our interpersonal interactions. I often think of my choir director constantly reminding us to be present in the room and to minimize distractions.

The 'R' stands for **'RESPONSIVENESS'** and will encourage us to reflect on our encounters and to keenly observe others so that we may adapt to changing scenarios and respond to cues that we are receiving during the encounters.

Through reflection, we can see how our perceptions and sometimes biases and experiences color our interactions with people around us and in response, we can alter our behaviors intentionally and perhaps better handle future interactions.

This may even be a good time to reflect on how your encounters and other scenarios are affecting you and to monitor and take note of the responses that they elicit from you, both negative and positive.

Responsiveness speaks to your immediate response to cues that you may receive during an individual encounter. These cues may immediately influence your behavior.

Reflection, on the other hand, draws on the need to take a broader look at how you tend to react and respond to varying cues and scenarios that lead to a more sustained change in behavior. It implies observing your past behaviors and attitudes over a longer period of time, and recognizing that there may be areas that need addressing.

The 'E' stands for **'ENGAGEMENT'** the need to be actually present and actively participating in the encounters.

When we are truly engaged we can better relate to patients and can navigate unfamiliar situations more effectively and comfortably.

As we grow through these power steps, we can begin to see a transformation in the way that we conduct ourselves as physicians and as humans in general.

## *A Personal Journey*

One of the most powerful aspects of the experience of authoring this book was the realization that I was writing a book to many versions of myself.

The exploration of the themes, issues, and concepts in this book addressed many of the struggles that I have either had, currently have, or anticipate that I will face in the future. What was even more powerful was the realization that I could help someone else who was feeling what I was feeling or who is going through what I was going through.

I honestly wish that I had read this book two decades ago. When you go through something and allow yourself to grow through it, it opens the door for you to be able to usher others through and make their path a little easier. This is truly giving back.

The struggles and pressures that we face as doctors can isolate us, but it is so comforting to know that someone out there may be feeling what you feel and may have insight that might help you navigate a situation.

It might be enough just to know that you are not alone and that behind many of the smiling faces that you encounter each day are others working through struggles just like you are, and those who made it despite the struggles. One of the benefits of success is the joy of showing others how to do it.

## *The Complexity of Doctoring*

As we consider the power steps to doctoring with a human touch, it can be so overwhelming. Honestly, Doctoring in and of itself is a scary thing. It is so fulfilling, but it is not without its inherent level of anxiety, nor should it be.

A certain small level of anxiety and commitment may help to 'keep you on your toes', but persistent and unchecked stress can lead to adverse effects. It is important that as physicians, and people constantly exposed to stressful situations, we find ways to manage this stress.

As we take on more responsibility in our roles, and as our lives evolve, it can be helpful to develop and discover tools and resources that can help us to simplify our lives.

Navigating a career, hopes, dreams, families, potential liability and all of the other facets of life can leave one feeling very vulnerable, and as we advance, the concerns that demand our attention and that tax us emotionally change.

Many of these concerns go unspoken, unaddressed, and undivulged.

## *Empowering Through Shared Experiences*

Through shared experiences, I hope that this writing can reach you at your point of need and help to pull or push you through whatever corridor you may find yourself in at the time of your reading.

These Power Steps on Doctoring with a Human Touch are meant to be a ubiquitously helpful tool for you as you navigate life as a doctor and provider of care. We are often seen only as Doctors and often the needs that we have go neglected.

As we become overwhelmed by our work and career, we can often lose touch with ourselves, our needs, our patients, and the reason that we first desired such a career.

Being burned out and tired can even cause us to lose the ability to communicate effectively and empathetically because we are simply trying to get through the day as quickly as possible.

## *A Reminder of Our Core Values*

Through the power steps outlined below, I want to remind you that the POWER to have an effective and fulfilling career and life is within reach. I hope that the tools in this book will help you to excel and to find peace in your career and your life.

As you Power through your day, just stop and remember these Important STEPS; Compassion, Awareness, Responsiveness, and Engagement.

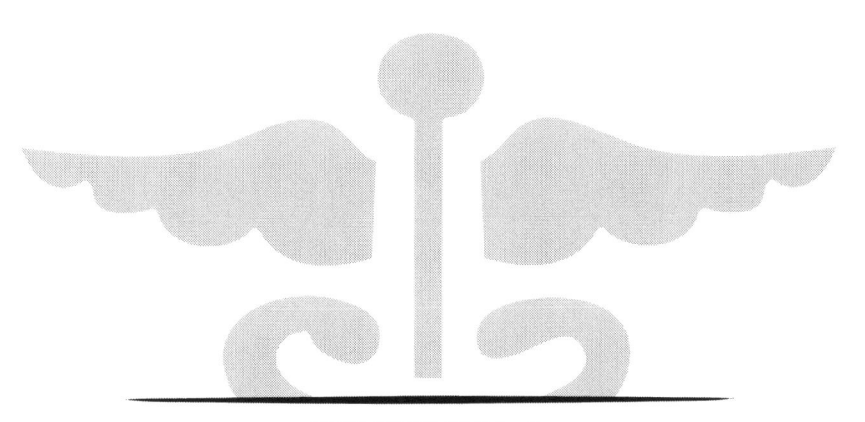

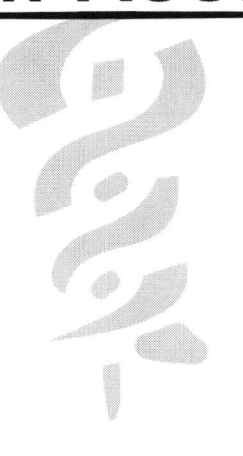

# SECTION 1
# COMPASSION

# COMPASSION

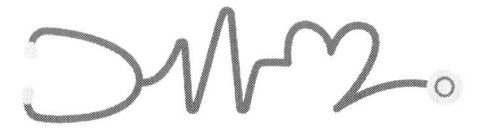

### "As you RACE through your Day, Don't Forget to C.A.R.E."

### "C" is for COMPASSION

One of the first steps to doctoring with a human touch is to remember the importance of compassion. Compassion speaks to the expression of concern about what others are experiencing.

In this section, we will discuss the roles that several power steps play in building our capacity to show and experience compassion, even when we may not feel inclined to do so.

I acknowledge, that despite considering myself a very compassionate person, it can be challenging to manifest this quality at the end of a long clinic day, or at 3 AM during an overnight shift when I am running on little rest. A serving of compassion, under these circumstances, can seem a daunting task.

I recall times when I had to retreat to a bathroom or another quiet place to take a moment and remind myself that this too shall pass. I would realize that the person seeking help does not know what I am going through; they are merely looking for assistance.

I might say out loud, "Let's go, Parker, we can do this," or sometimes, I would scream quietly or stomp in frustration. These thirty-nine-second pep talks or moments of release allowed me to regroup and 'get on with the show.'

It's crucial to discover what works for you so that you can employ the strategy that best helps you navigate these tough moments.

In this section, we will dissect and perfect three of the power steps, namely: The Power of Compassion, The Power of Being Human and Vulnerable, and The Power of Acknowledgment.

I want to emphasize from the outset that compassion for yourself, though not frequently discussed, is absolutely mandatory!

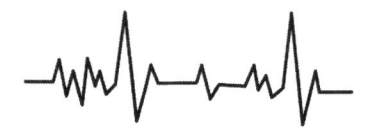

# Chapter 1

# The Power of Compassion

Compassion and vulnerability are not mutually exclusive with professionalism in medicine, or in any other profession really. When I think of compassion, I think of showing genuine concern for the well-being of someone else, and seeking to do something to help them.

Compassion is relatively easy to develop in interpersonal relationships with those with whom we have developed close bonds, and it is relatively easy to show in these scenarios. It's easy to cry with a sister or a best friend when something goes wrong, and you don't consciously think about your vulnerability being plainly on display.

## *The Challenge of Vulnerability in Medicine*

To be vulnerable, and to be emotionally or otherwise exposed, is so fragile a state of existence that it tends to be generally avoided, when possible, in the practice of medicine, and perhaps in most other social situations. Now, this is not always the case, and this is certainly not intended to suggest that physicians and health care professionals in general are, by nature, cold and unemotional or disconnected.

In fact, the converse tends to be true, and in general, people tend to be drawn to the practice of medicine because it puts them in a position to help people. This is obviously not the only reason to pursue a career in medicine, but it certainly helps to check the 'fulfillment' box when choosing a career.

## *Emotional Availability and Its Limits*

There can be advantages to budgeting your emotional availability when it comes to patient interactions. Let's face it, we can't cry 40 times per day, this would be both inefficient and quite emotionally and physically taxing. Besides, I think we ourselves would be referred for some sort of professional evaluation as constant crying would not fit into societal norms.

So, in a professional space where we are sometimes repeatedly exposed to pain, sickness, loss, hurt, stress, death, trauma, abuse, and despair; while being expected to think objectively, listen attentively, interpret physical examinations and investigations accurately, and make sound (and correct) clinical judgments, we can appear somewhat emotionally disconnected as we maintain our composure, and lead the medical team, and the patient, and the family in the decision-making process.

## *The Unseen Struggles of Healthcare Professionals*

What the patients don't see are the tears that the doctor cries in the bathroom when she witnesses a child dying as the mother sits helplessly at the bedside. What they don't see is the lonely midnight drive home while the doctor is going over every single event and lab value with a fine-toothed comb, wondering if there is something else that could be done to change the odds.

What they don't see is the marriage that is strained because the doctor can't seem to keep her emotional attachment and distress about the goings on of her workday out of her mind when she gets home to her husband and children.

What they don't see is the 17 phone calls (both the necessary and the unnecessary) to the doctor overnight while he is being updated with every clinical change of his patient in the ICU. What they don't see is the house call at 2 AM to officially pronounce the death of a long-time patient who had now become a friend. What they don't see is the trauma experienced by the intern when he conducts his first 'code' and loses his first patient!

He thinks to himself, 'But we are in the hospital, we did everything according to the recommended protocol, we gave the medications and counted the compressions and did everything 'right', but still, my patient died! What do I say to his family?'.

What they don't see is the tears the resident sheds because she has missed both the wedding of her best friend and the funeral of her closest cousin because she couldn't get someone to cover her ICU call.

What they don't see is the doctor who just had a miscarriage after her overnight shift, which was followed by a clinic the following morning (in places where this still happens). What they don't see is the heartbreak of the doctor who delivers a stillborn baby for a woman who has lost 4 prior pregnancies and we don't know why.

What they don't see is that the doctor is actually petrified of something going 'wrong'; because in the midst of all the charged emotions, compassion, and empathy that he might be experiencing, things can, and do go wrong!

The things that can go wrong are so many ...and sometimes not related to the actual action or inaction of the physician... BUT...when they do go wrong... just like that...everyone looks at him and says. 'YOU SHOULD HAVE...!'

The doctor should have known this... or should have done that... or should have seen this coming... or should have known that the patient would have had an allergic reaction to a random drug. The doctor should have predicted this outcome or warned the family of that particular outcome.

It's amazing that the doctor functions at all... knowing that even the nicest of patients could 'turn on him' with blame, litigation, and condemnation if something were to 'go wrong'. Let's not even get started on what could happen in the 'court' of social media.

Patients make their own decisions and can have idiosyncratic reactions and simply just have a bad outcome just because they had a bad outcome... but none of that matters in the eyes of the patient, the family, and in the eyes of those who are quick to judge.

Medicine is one of the few professions where everything is expected to go right and where the practitioner is blamed for things that are sometimes beyond his ability to control.

We are not referring to cases of absolute irresponsibility or obvious negligence, but in general, this is a high-stakes profession and medicine is a very jealous mistress.

She often can take first place if you let her and if you fear consequences and judgment, she can take over your conscious and subconscious being also. You can live in constant fear of what you forgot to do or of what you did that could be perceived as having been done incorrectly, or of what you did that was actually less than ideal.

You could be constantly petrified of the possibility of a result coming in that you didn't see yet or of not receiving the result at all, especially if the patient decided that it was not important enough to keep the follow-up appointment where the results of the tests would have been reviewed and discussed. This is very serious.

The practice of medicine is truly a calling and it's truly scary. Many continue to judge the service that physicians provide as inadequate. They are failing to realize that sometimes there are restrictions based on the availability of resources and the presence of bureaucratic dogma and the burden of excessive patient loads.

The physician is one of the only professionals who is expected to be infallible and function with a 'zero tolerance' for errors. The physician is not God, he is not all-knowing but he is expected to practice as such.

Many walk away from the profession because of the unrelenting pressure. Being compassionate can be so difficult when one is practicing defensively, but amidst all the pressure of practicing medicine, one must still find it within oneself to show compassion.

## *Coping Mechanisms and the Imperative of Compassion*

So, having had to cope with all the adjustments that one must encounter as one journeys through university then medical school, then postgraduate training with residencies and fellowships as directed by choice of specialty, one tends to develop certain mechanisms to cope with the range of emotional and physical experiences encountered on this journey. This can lead us to tend toward a very tempered emotional connection with our patients.

And to be honest, this will suffice for most clinical interactions and will likely be appropriate for most of those physician-patient relationships.

## *Building a Deeper Connection*

The challenge will be to recognize those times when, though stretched, it is both appropriate and necessary to allow a deeper emotional connection between yourself and your patient. And this does not always necessarily speak to an outward display of emotional vulnerability. This can be as simple as speaking to a patient in the 'dialect' that they are familiar with if there is one, and if you know it, and you are a part of their culture. This can be the one time that the patient feels that they have connected with the true and authentic you.

This can also allow them to feel that they can display themselves and all their vulnerabilities and sometimes this opens the door to secrets that unlock the door to hidden concerns that the patient has not voiced, despite having seen multiple physicians before coming to you. This can sometimes be the one bit of information that makes the mystery diagnosis plainly clear, because they have let you into the 'circle of trust' and divulged the one piece of the puzzle that completes the diagnostic picture and 'connects the dots'.

## The Transformative Power of Compassionate Care

I remember seeing an elderly patient once at a clinic. He was being seen by me for management of his diabetes, so of course, I took a history, examined this patient, and reviewed his current medications, which he had brought to the visit.

I was so appreciative of him bringing his medications to the visit. We went on to review his labs and I made only a few adjustments to his medications because his diabetes control was not particularly suboptimal given his age and comorbidities.

So, nearing the end of the interview, he held his head down and said that he wanted to ask about something and that he was not sure that he should or could ask.

I responded to him that if there was something that was concerning to him, he certainly should ask about it, and if it was not something that I could effectively address I may be able to initiate the evaluation and then refer him to someone more equipped to address the concern.

This patient went on to ask if there was anything that could be done because he was having difficulty with his libido and his erections. I told him that many factors contribute to the achievement of an erection, that we could certainly start the evaluation for those things, and that if there was anything that was obviously deficient, like perhaps a testosterone deficiency, then we could do the requisite evaluation and proceed to treatment.

I also advised him that a urology consultation would be initiated after the initial lab evaluation and that there was a distinct possibility that there was meaningful help available for his condition. I told him that the quality of his life was just as important as the quantity of his life, and that if there was something that could be done to improve it, I believed that we should do it.

So, we made a plan for labs and ultrasound and a plan to follow up in two weeks to review the results and make the intervention as appropriate. I stood and gave him a gentle pat on the shoulder and reassured him that we would do our best to help him.

His response nearly floored me. It didn't, but it nearly did! This patient held his head down and began to sob inconsolably. He cried for what seemed like several minutes and I stood by his side and waited silently.

I may have passed him a tissue but at this moment I can't recall if I did that or not. When he managed to gather his composure, he looked me in the eye for a few moments as if to say something. So, I looked back and smiled and asked him what was going on and what had upset him.

He looked down toward his lap (he was sitting) and continued to look down as he said to me that he was crying because he was overwhelmed that someone 'like me' would spend so much time and effort to take care of and help 'someone like him'.

I said to him, why wouldn't I take care of you, that's why I'm here and I proceeded to escort him to the door so that that coordinator could assist him with making his follow-up appointment.

He was from a southern state in the United States of America, so I will leave it to your imagination what he meant by 'someone like you' and 'someone like me'.

## *Compassion Beyond Boundaries*

The bottom line is, that being compassionate in the way you relate to someone can sometimes have an impact that is far more powerful than you could have ever imagined.

You could be impacting generational experiences and stereotypes and healing personal turmoil so deeply that it literally changes someone. It could even change you.

You can be thorough, accurate, exceptional, and correct, but imagine being all that and also being NICE!

Though compassion is most beautiful and revered, if you observe her closely enough, she may appear not only to be blind, but also deaf, and amnestic.

She gives no credence to race, sex, gender, age, religion, spirituality, nationality, past wrongdoings, culture, smell, ethnicity, socioeconomic status, size, weight, or any other thing that may seek to distract her.

There are so many 'isms' that may consciously or subconsciously influence how we view the world and how others view us. In addition, there are 'isms' that influence someone's expectations of us.

We have to make a special effort to be aware of our vulnerability to such influences, as they may impact us; either as recipients of premature judgment based on something as irrelevant as our race or gender; or as perpetrators of such injustices, based for example, on the age of a patient or his apparent economic status or his weight.

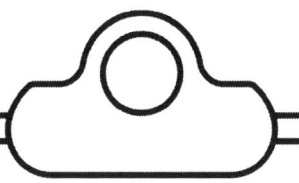

## BOTTOM LINE

Allow yourself to be compassionate and to show it, even if only in small ways.

# ℞ ACTION PLAN

- [ ] Think of phrases that you can interject into your clinical encounters that can express compassion. This is important if you tend to go out of your way to maintain your distance, and to be super-fast and efficient. Phrases like, 'I can see why this is difficult for you' or 'This is truly a lot ma'am, take your time' can help you to show compassion.

- [ ] Try to stay away from phrases like 'I totally understand', because you probably don't (unless of course, you do!).

# The Power of Compassion

***Part 2: Cultivating Compassion Among Colleagues***

The trek through medical school and the intense training that happens thereafter is a tough one. On our journey along this path, we will encounter many whose lives we will influence and who will influence us.

As we work to survive, and if we're lucky, to thrive in a very tough, demanding, and competitive environment, let us not forget the power of compassion for each other.

We are trained from the outset that medicine is cutthroat (no pun intended, ENT docs), and competitive, and we all know the proverbial (or for some literal) introduction to medical school, where someone stands afront the audience of eager medical students and says these words: 'look to your left and look to your right, one of these persons will not make it to graduation with you!'

And from the outset, these people are your competition. I thought that the competition was to get into medical school, I didn't realize that I now had to compete again.

But whether by nature or by training, medical students perhaps tend to be more competitive than most. Perhaps that proverbial speech is meant to motivate you to put your head into your books and to get the job done.

Statistically speaking, I do believe that the graduation rate of students entering medical school is generally in excess of 90% in some instances. This may not be the case everywhere, but it is certainly encouraging.

So, guess what guys, we're probably going to make it. And we all know the old joke right, 'what do you call the medical student that graduated at the bottom of the class?...Doctor!' ...Exactly.

## *Competing with Myself and Embracing Failure*

Now, I cannot state that I was immune to a sense of competition while journeying through medical school. I would have to say that there was always a healthy sense of competition and camaraderie. However, I always was, and remain, deep in competition with myself.

I never really felt pressure to beat anyone or to come first or second. I simply had, and probably still have, a deep fear of failure. Many of us do. Entrepreneurs and the like are the people, in my experience, who have mastered their relationships with failure. They use what we call 'failure' as a chance to pivot and improve.

If this idea doesn't work, they clean up the mess (or not), and move on to the next great idea, sometimes taking what worked from the last business attempt, and sometimes trying something entirely new. They have a completely different connection with failure than we are trained or conditioned to have.

For us, failure is not an option. Now, for someone who has had three generations of family members including aunties, uncles, grandparents, and cousins, all working as laborers to cover the cost of college and then medical school, this may seem to be true.

Perhaps he or she is the first one to go to college ever, and the thought of death may pale in comparison to the thought of returning to the family having 'failed out' of medical school.

The thing is, we don't necessarily know who is carrying such a burden, but the truth is that someone may be. So, we must remember, as medical students, that the majority of us will indeed graduate, and that those who are stronger can serve as sources of inspiration and motivation for those of us who are weaker.

I treasure the few friends that I made during my course of training. Most people will make friends and find study groups, but remember to look out for the ones that seem to not quite fit in.

A kind word or an invitation for companionship may save someone's life or at the very least, may influence their future or their willingness to continue. Admittedly, these are lessons that might have served me well while I was in training. It takes nothing from you to be nice to someone. The hard part was getting in.

One source[1] cites that overall, about 43% of applicants to osteopathic medical schools in the U.S. were accepted for 2022-2023. Individual medical schools can have acceptance rates from just over 1% to just under 9%.[2,3] This number, of course, can vary significantly depending on the location of the medical school, with some medical schools accepting a significantly higher percentage of applicants. Furthermore, most medical students graduate from medical school!

So, you're in. Make friends, these people will be your colleagues and you will share memories with them, or at least some of them, for the rest of your life. I hope that you get the chance to connect with at least a few of them.

### *Nurturing Environments and Future Leaders*

Now, while most medical schools provide a very nurturing environment, are very supportive of students, and are vested in the well-being and success of their enrollees, it is important, when you are in a position of authority, that you remember that you were once like these people and that these people will become you one day.

Ask yourself... when they become you, who will you be? This goes for every stage of the training process. Try to remain grounded, no matter the height to which you may ascend and how accomplished you may become.

Remember to be encouraging and to contribute, if only in small ways, to these people who want so much to be like who they perceive you to be. You are uniquely positioned to be a positive influence or to be a negative one.

If you live in a small enough place, one of them may be your doctor one day as you lay demented on the ward, having once stood as a leader in your field.

## *Standing on the Shoulders of Mentors*

I stand on the shoulders of many mentors, both living and not, who poured into me as a school student, university student, medical student, resident, fellow, and early career physician.

I remember eagerly following them around and attending after-school lectures and tutorials. I remember waking up on Saturday mornings to attend exam preparation classes and lectures. I remember residents taking us under their wings and going through cases with us and reviewing topics with us.

I remember attendings and consultants giving me articles to read, and I remember reading every single one of them, marking and cross-referencing them, and color coding them... matching pens and highlighters and all! I remember being challenged on ward rounds and preparing myself to do more than answer questions the following day.

And if they forgot to ask me, I would remind them that I had something to talk about or I would find a way to integrate it into the answer for another question. I remember literally running after an attending to make sure he knew that we were ready for ward rounds and teaching (lol, yep...that was me).

I remember being brought to literal tears on ward rounds one fine morning because I felt so pressured when asked a question in front of the team. I knew the answer and gave it, but somehow I became overwhelmed by the moment and bawled like something happened to me.

I remember it all as if it were yesterday, and my resident at the time (who is now a well-established and respected consultant physician) remembers it too...lol.

I remember being coached before final practical exams by consultants (attendings) in the halls leading up to the patient exam stations...saying words like 'Reach for the moon Parker, and if you somehow miss...you will at least land somewhere amongst the stars'. These were reminders that I was well prepared for what lay ahead.

It was as if we were in the locker room and about to make our entrance onto the field for the final game of the playoffs...and they were squirting sports drinks in my mouth through the shield grill of my helmet and misting my forehead with water...really it was a breath mint...and there were no sports drinks or spray fans...but you get my point.

I found a team of mentors that gave and gave and gave, and I am eternally grateful for the sacrifices that they made for us. They gave of their time, their money, and their lives just to shape us, and if any of them are reading this book, they know exactly who they are.

They showed ultimate compassion, they treated us like family, like children really, and they literally built us; one lecture and one tutorial, one kind word, and one extra class at a time.

## *Facing Challenges and Embracing Compassion*

While this journey has been undeniably gracious to me, I have had the distinct pleasure of coming across a few who have been intimidating and inconsiderate towards me or my colleagues.

Many can become obstructionists and unwelcoming forces who tend to see young doctors as competition as opposed to succession engineers. This may be a cultural phenomenon or perhaps a function of operating in a smaller society.

This, in fact, may not be unique to medicine. But fortunately, I grew up in a place where the people 'in charge' on many levels looked like me, and in some scenarios, were known to me or knew me or were even related to me.

So, I always had trouble seeing someone or some title or some achievement as being out of my reach. I always figured that if I really wanted to do something, that I, or someone with whom I have been in contact, could probably do it.

By this, I mean that I always just saw 'Senior Doctors' as people who happened to be born before I was and therefore, they were doctors before I was ... so this chasm that some would try to create between themselves and their 'juniors' always seemed false and fickle.

I wondered if they realized that they would get older and weaker just like everyone else would if they were lucky. Did they realize that they could have a heart attack or stroke just like anyone could?

Did they realize that I know that they pee and poop and fart just like me and that we were not that different after all...truly, I believe that some of them did not at that time realize that.

What am I saying? I'm saying to be compassionate to people, even those who are 'beneath you.' They will soon be above you!! Train them well. You can't be in your position forever! It's a distinct impossibility.

## *Facing Misguided Opinions with Determination*

I remember being asked by an authority figure what I was going to specialize in. I will always remember this 'senior' doctor's flippant response to me, which was...'WASTE OF TIME!'

Yes, in a world where diabetes, obesity, and chronic non-communicable diseases are rampant and devastating, a budding endocrinologist was advised that studying endocrinology was a waste of time. Getting a fellowship in endocrinology was no easy task, but that is another story for another day.

## *Cultivating Self-Compassion and Resilience*

Guard your words and guard your hearts. Not everyone remembers to be humble and compassionate, so you must remember to be compassionate to yourself. You know what you are capable of, and you know what gifts God placed within you. You must manifest your unique greatness and pour out of it into the world.

While, as in my experience, most will go out of their way to help you, and the universe will make room for you and your gifts,[4] guard your heart against those who seek not to build you up, but only to pull you down[5]. Remember to speak positively and optimistically to others and yourself.

You never know who is on 'the brink' and remember to reach out if it is you that needs the help.

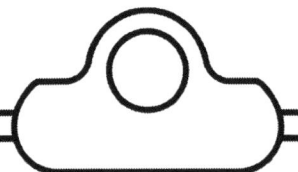

## BOTTOM LINE

Remember that those around you may need a kind word.

Remember that most of you will graduate from medical school. Be kind to others, even those not as popular as you are.

Remember that those looking up to you may soon be looking down at you as you lay in the patient bed and they stand in the white coat.

# ℞ ACTION PLAN

- [ ] The next time you come across a medical student, resident, consultant, attending or colleague as you go about your duties, ask them if they are ok, and actually listen to the answer. Sometimes, that was all that was needed.

- [ ] Think twice before you say something demeaning or hurtful to someone.

# The Power of Compassion

### PART 3: SELF-COMPASSION: THE FOUNDATION OF CAREGIVING

In the section before this one, I briefly touched on the tip of the iceberg of emotional experiences that someone in the practice of medicine can experience, to some degree or another, daily.

The day-to-day welfare of the physician is seldom the primary concern of the patient, the family, the medical system, the staff, or even the physician. We regularly work long hours and fail to prepare proper meals for ourselves.

Many of us eat poorly, utilize drive-throughs, are overweight, and are in poor general health. Most of us don't meet the minimum exercise recommendations that are recommended for our patients and for society at large.

Medicine is demanding. From the moment that one considers pursuing a career in medicine, it shapes their life. They start engaging in extracurricular activities because they want to be more 'well-rounded' to appear as more attractive applicants to medical schools.

Many people are engaged in such activities out of sheer interest, but once they start considering this career path, they make sure that they get involved in things outside of academics.

This, of course, assumes that they, at the same time, will maintain a stellar academic record. Being above average just won't do, and so the pressure is on!

I feel sorry for those who knew that they wanted to be doctors since high school because for those people, the pressure began long before it should have. The need to be better, or the best, is an insane one that can push one to great levels of achievement and stress.

The undergraduate experience, if this is the track that you take, is also pressured, and focused on achievements over experiences. In some systems, you do 'A' Levels rather than an undergraduate degree, so your life experience is tailored only for academia and the rigors of competitiveness.

Once in medical school, you are tasked with finishing medical school and trying to secure your spot in your desired area of postgraduate specialization, if you have one.

Alternatively, you are trying to get accepted into anything quite frankly. If you do not have a plan, then you can find yourself in a very peculiar situation. All of this is to say that once you have decided that medicine is your desired career path, it can be all-consuming.

All who are physicians know what they have been through, and all who have married, parented, lived with, been siblings to, close relatives of, or best friends to aspiring physicians, and have observed them on their journey, can bear witness to the fact that the journey is not one for the weak, and that in general, the journey ends in more work and more commitment, and even more sacrifice.

I remember the true story of a surgical resident who asked for a day off about 9 months in advance, so that he could have his wedding on that date. This date also worked for his fiancé, who was a resident in another program nearby. In response to his request, which was denied, he was advised that the schedule was set and that he should learn to plan his life around his work schedule, and not his work schedule around his life. And here again, we see perfectly illustrated, how demanding and unforgiving the practice of medicine can be.

I remember another story of a resident, who only weeks after losing his sibling in an accident, was advised that he needed to adjust quickly, as the call schedule was not going to accomodate him forever. And while this may be true, that does not make it any less harsh a reality.

## *A Reminder to Live and Care for Yourself*

Dear doctor, you have been through so much to get to this point, and it is so easy for us to forget to live. It is so easy for us to lend compassion to others and to forget to do so to ourselves. It is so easy to give until we have nothing else.

We are susceptible to burnout, depression, physical illness, and mental illness, just like everyone else.[1] We need someone to remind us to take care of ourselves. We forget so often that if we die, they will hire someone else to fill our position yesterday!

Our patients will find another doctor. They may miss you, but they are their number one priority. Consider making yourself a priority too!

Be compassionate to yourself! Be kind to yourself! Remember to live while you are training. Go to the Broadway show! See the movie! Take the trip! Go to the ball game... even if you're a little tired.

Read the book, for pleasure, one page at a time, because we all know that time is the one thing that we don't have much of to spare and, the one thing that we can't get back.

Watch the show! Cry! Get your hair done! Get your nails done! Take the day off! Get the pap smear and mammogram! Get the colonoscopy! You're tired, go to the doctor! It might be something serious. It CAN happen to you! Look out for yourself. Get counseling. Join the group or the club. Take the tour.

Find the things in life that make you happy and do them! Build yourself up mentally, spiritually, psychologically, financially, physically, emotionally!! You must have something in your cup if you expect to have something to pour into others. If you are empty, from whence are you giving?

Even Jesus himself withdrew into the protective cape of solitude, on multiple occasions to recharge, to grieve, to pray, to pause before making important decisions, and for other reasons.[2]

Even God rested on the 7th day of creation[3]. It is not selfish to take care of yourself. It's mandatory. Find your quiet place, find YOUR source, and go to it regularly to be filled. If you burn your candle from both ends, there is no doubt in my mind, that you will experience the inevitable 'Burn out'!

## *Finding Balance: Living Through the Journey*

When young people would ask me 'How did you stay in school so long?' I didn't have a satisfactory answer for them, because I had never thought about it. I have met more than a few people who said they wanted to be doctors but felt it would take too long and therefore they could not pursue such a career path.

I learned to answer this question after some introspection, and the answer is, that while I was in medical school, I lived. While I was in residency and fellowship, I lived. I enjoyed my environment, tried to stay involved, and enjoyed where I lived while I was there.

Of course, hindsight is 20/20, and if I had known then what I now know, I would have done even more at each stage of my training. The funny thing about time is that it will pass by regardless of what you choose to do, and at the end of a certain period of time (however long it is), you either would have done what you wanted to do, or you wouldn't have.

So, I decided to do what I wanted to do, and the time passed...as time does...and what I said I would do, was done.

## *Self-Compassion: The Foundation of Caregiving*

So, here is some advice that I might have done well with if someone had given it to me: in all the doing, do for you! In all the giving, give to you. In all the loving, love you. In all the praying, pray for you.

In all the caring, care for you. In all the advising, save some for yourself. When you are healthy and happy and strong and whole, you can continue to give of yourself to the degree that you are called so to do.

## *Self-Care Is Not Selfish: Embracing Your Own Needs*

'First, do no harm'...Did it ever occur to you that this applies to you, in the care that you offer to yourself? We give to and care for others, but the truth is, many of us really don't take the time to see ourselves as ones in need of caring.

Patients call, they email, they message, they show up, they make appointments, they skip them, they demand answers and responses, and sometimes they expect more of you than they do of themselves.

Some would say 'If you didn't want to serve, then why did you choose a career in medicine?' Some people are ruthless in their view of physicians and feel that they deserve your care and attention, no matter what!

Some believe that it is somehow your duty to care for them, even when they have failed to care for themselves, for years, and are now faced with the complications, and manifestations of that lack of caring.

The pressure is on you! The pressure can be relentless. You are the DOCTOR! Fix it...or else!! And they better not die; and don't let anything happen to their relative!!

They come after you because, after all, it was not the alcohol, the smoking, the disease, the stress, the lack of proper nutrition and exercise that caused this to happen to them, it was you. The moment 'something happens' all of a sudden, they come for you!

## The Misconceptions About Being a Physician

Some are of the view that doctors go into medicine to make a lot of money. Many physicians can become legitimately wealthy in the practice of medicine, depending on the specialty and other factors, including business acumen and investment portfolio, but the majority don't.

Many physicians don't have the financial acumen to end their careers as wealthy individuals and should, in fact, consider some financial coaching.

The hours worked and the decades of life dedicated to qualifying as a physician make many other career choices significantly more lucrative and far better choices than medicine if one was truly in it solely to make money.

Some are resentful of physicians because of their perceived or actual wealth, but there is so much more to being a physician, so much that was lost and sacrificed in the process. So much that those who envy you would refuse to sacrifice themselves.

You have given of yourself in ways that truly only others who have sacrificed this way will really understand. Yes, there are some that do egregious things in the name of medicine, to make money and even do harm to patients in the process.

But these are not the majority, and these are not the physicians about whom we are speaking. Take the time to rest, rebuild, recharge, rejuvenate, and revitalize yourself. It's ok to need it.

## Beyond Medicine: Finding Meaning and Purpose

Many physicians die soon after retirement.

Many have done nothing outside of medicine, and when the opportunity to practice their craft is taken away, by retirement, by age, by being replaced, by injury or illness, and by many other things, they find themselves unable to truly integrate into society in a way that brings meaning to themselves.

They sacrificed relationships and connections, sometimes to those most dependent on, and important to them. While their service above self was appreciated, and undoubtedly had significant impacts on the patients and communities that they served, they did nothing else to enrich their lives and to allow them to find a personal sense of meaning outside of medicine.

This is so easy to do. It is so easy to work from sun-up to sun-down and to feel so needed by others now, that you fail to see that you were needed by your own being. Your mindfulness about your needs, both present and future, was needed while you were in your 'prime'.

So, now that the future is the present, you realize that your investment solely in the past has robbed you of your usefulness to yourself in your current present.

Be involved in things outside of your practice. Keep up with family and friends. Join a club. Acknowledge that you need nurturing and social integration, no matter how small it is.

Doctors are seen by others, and often by themselves, to be somewhat invincible in a way. We do not often consider what it would be like to be a patient. Others don't often imagine that their doctors are someone else's patients, that they have their own diagnoses to grapple with sometimes, and that they have their own struggles.

Many don't care really. You are there to serve them. We often don't see ourselves in that role either. Some of us have a fear of what would be there if we checked. We know too much, it's scary out there. Many of us don't make the time to check.

It is not infrequent for me to see one of my patients sitting in the waiting room at the doctor's office where I am also in the waiting room, waiting to see the doctor. They never fail to look at me as if to ask why I am at a doctor's office.

I remember talking to a colleague about something as simple as going to the eye doctor. I remember seeing her wearing glasses one day and I commented about how academic and stately she looked and asked her when she started wearing glasses.

She began to share how for months she would be watching television and assuming that the words were blurry for everyone when closed captioning was on, or when there was a commercial playing. She talked about having headaches sometimes and would take a painkiller. Someone at her office eventually suggested that she get her eyes checked, and so she did.

She looked at me and said, 'You know it's strange because I just never thought that something could happen to me! It just never occurred to me that something could happen to ME!'

Now, this was fortunately quite an inconsequential happening, but many of us tend to be and are also trained to be oblivious to our own needs. It is seriously frowned upon to miss work, to miss rounds, to call in sick, or to not perform during your training.

You could easily be typecast as lazy, weak, uncommitted, unintelligent, not up to snuff or just not cut out to be a doctor. Being tired, sick, sad, or overwhelmed are definitely things that you hide, and learn to mask and cope with.

Complainers aren't going to be very popular interns or residents, and to be perceived as such, can make life difficult for you. Efficiency and dedication are king, and anything that compromises your ability to be any of these things can land you being labeled, or even worse, ostracized during your training.

We become very good at gritting and grinding and making it happen. Check that box! Get the list done! No matter what!

This fortitude clearly has its role, considering your eventual role as a physician, and one who is depended upon during people's most vulnerable moments, but it comes at a cost.

## *Breaking the Stigma: Mental Health in the Medical Profession*

For fear of appearing weak or appearing as one not able to cope with the rigors of medicine, it would be my guess, that more than just a few physicians would decline seeking help from a mental health professional.

There was, and is a stigma, in general communities, and within the fraternity of medicine, about persons requiring help for their mental health.

This, in my perception, is getting significantly better through the work of awareness campaigns and because of the sheer commonness of the mental health concerns and ailments that affect people.

Many of us now know someone affected by mental illness or someone who decided to seek therapy to discuss issues that might be affecting them.

Because people are becoming more open about having therapists, and because it's now commonly depicted on the big screen, and because people now bring it up in conversation, there might be more of a willingness of doctors to seek the help of a mental health professional or to at least recognize that they need to talk to someone.

This can even start out as 'opening up' to a close friend, family member, or religious leader. 'Opening up' and talking about an issue is one of the first steps to healing because talking about something forces us to acknowledge that there is indeed something that needs talking about and addressing.

Physicians are at increased risk for successful suicide acts compared to other professionals and the general population, so we must look out for ourselves and for others.

We CAN be our brother's keepers. We can pull someone aside and say that it will be ok, we can reach out to the weakest intern in the class and give them a word of motivation.

Who knows what personal struggles someone carries along with them on their journey through life and through medicine. A kind and encouraging word may be the difference between someone's sense of hope and someone's decision to commit an act that would create a permanent end to their life or career in response to a stressor that was transient.

Sometimes we need to be reminded that 'this too shall pass'. Don't underestimate the impact that you can have on someone else's life.

Being positive and encouraging is also 'self-therapeutic'. It is very difficult to bring light to someone else while remaining completely engulfed in the darkness that is your own. The light that you give to someone will inevitably bring light to you!

Talk to someone about what you are going through. Your willingness to be vulnerable may save a life that may well be your own.

The fear of rejection can cause someone to hold tight to experiences and feelings, that if expressed and addressed, could change the trajectory of their entire life. We fear being deemed unfit to practice the craft to which we have dedicated so much of ourselves, our time, our lives, and our reproductive potential.

We reject the idea of possible rejection, and we put ourselves at risk for losing our very own lives. This is your permission ticket to accept that you are vulnerable, that you are sometimes in need of help, and that your feelings matter!

Your wellness is important, if not to anyone else, TO YOU!! You are a doctor! But for you to truly heal and pour into others, you must first, to yourself be true, be kind, and be considerate.

## *The Hard Work of Caring: The Emotional Labor of Physicians*

What many don't understand, is that caring is very hard work. Going the extra mile is exhausting. Walking on a health journey with a patient is physically and mentally draining and fatiguing.

Taking the time to research the symptoms of a patient, to come up with a list of differentials when someone does not quite fit the typical presentation is tiring. Being the one to try to figure something out after a patient has seen several specialists is daunting and taxing, and deciding to take on the challenge is not easy.

Often, the patient is impatient because this has been their struggle for many months and they have had many assessments, but this is the first time YOU have seen them, and the pressure and sometimes desperation that they feel is immediately palpable by you.

I once met a lady who had literally seen nine specialists while investigating her current complaint over the ensuing 11 months. I was the tenth doctor she was seeing for this complaint. The TENTH!

The pursuit of the well-being of your patient can be pervasive and can start to invade moments far away from the clinical setting. Trying to help someone and wanting to see them do well does not end when the clinical encounter ends, and your mind doesn't stop when the office closes or when the patient leaves the encounter.

No one can pay you for what it truly takes to take care of a patient, especially one that requires more than baseline care. The protective mechanisms that clinicians can sometimes employ to protect themselves from emotional burnout can make them seem detached, cold, and callous, but sometimes this is the result of many years of bleeding with your patients.

Becoming overwhelmed, especially in clinical settings where you are practicing with limited resources, can leave you wanting to do more for patients than you physically can. Sometimes restricted access to resources can limit your practice and interfere with the positive reinforcement that a sense of satisfaction brings.

Knowing what is ideal to offer a patient and knowing that they do not have access to this, for various reasons, is disheartening and can bring a sense of hopelessness, dissatisfaction, and frustration. These scenarios demand that you be as merciful to yourself as you are merciful to others.

Dearest doctor, take time for you! You are wonderful, powerful, intelligent, diligent, caring, and giving, and you seek perfection in all that you do. So much is required of you, and you give it, often without fail, and often at great cost. All this means that you are also in need of great love and that you deserve to have someone invest in YOU!!

Be your own someone!

Invest in yourself!

Give yourself the gift of self-love!!

Accept the love of others and of God.

This will help to empower you to continue to give and to serve to the best of your ability! When you find peace, this sense of balance emanates from you and causes others to seek to be around you.

A physician who brings a sense of peace and calm will attract many patients. So, rather than working solely on building your practice, work first on building yourself! The practice will seek you as you build it!!!

## *Empowerment Through Communication: A Path Forward*

Now that you have decided to add the skill of effective communication to your armamentarium, you will be even more equipped and empowered to excel and to continue to conquer new giants in your life.

Put into practice the nuggets of knowledge that you will pick up from this writing and get ready to move on to the next step in your journey of self-improvement.

There is a great communicator in you, and the world needs to hear your voice, one patient at a time!

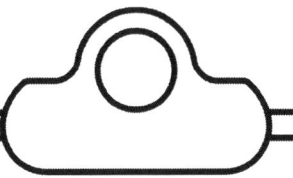

## BOTTOM LINE

It's mandatory to take care of yourself and to enjoy the one chance at life that you get. Be the recipient of your own compassion.

Invest in interests outside of your practice.

Go to the doctor and take care of yourself.

# ℞ ACTION PLAN

- [ ] Find one thing that you enjoy doing and do it at least once per week. It does not have to be big. It could be buying yourself a bouquet of flowers from the grocery store or bodega. If flowers make you happy, don't wish to receive them, buy them for yourself or pick them and put them in a vase on the table.

- [ ] If you love plays, don't wait to be invited, go see the play. Pay for someone to come with you if you really don't want to go alone. It's nice going alone, but that's just me.

- [ ] Take a walk for 30 minutes daily to clear your head and to exercise if you don't have a regular regimen. Your future will thank you when it becomes the present.

## Chapter 2

# The Power of Acknowledgement

As we work toward improving our ability to show compassion, it is important to remember the power of acknowledgment. There is nothing quite as powerful as walking into a patient's room and addressing them by their name.

Nothing beats being acknowledged. Is there anyone who does not appreciate being recognized, and enthusiastically so?

### *The Power of a Personal Greeting*

The first thing I do when I walk into a patient's room or when a patient walks into my office for a consultation is say their name.

"Good morning, Mrs. Brown! My name is Dr. Parker-Curling! To what do I owe this distinct pleasure???" Or "What brings us together today?"

Sometimes I'd say, "Are you the one and only Jo Black?" as I walked into the encounter, flashing the biggest smile while approaching them with an outstretched hand. Other times, I'd say, "To what do I owe this great pleasure, honor, privilege, and challenge?" Just observe the patient and the mood and make what you think is the appropriate introduction.

## *Navigating Miscommunication and Ensuring Correct Identification*

Be careful, though. It is astonishing how many patients will smile and nod to the wrong name and sometimes go along with the story. This can be especially true when mask-wearing adds a physical barrier to communication and can cause a person to mishear.

Sometimes it's even wise to say, "Am I in the room of Mrs. White?" or perhaps you can try "Whom do I have the pleasure of meeting today?" Or you can say, "Good afternoon, my name is Dr. Gray. What is your name?" and take it from there. Sometimes simple is best.

## *Building a Therapeutic Relationship Through Acknowledgment*

Immediately, the response from the patient is nothing but a smile! Even in the most somber of encounters, acknowledging a patient by their name opens the door to communication and to the potential of a long (or sometimes short) and healthy therapeutic relationship that can pave the way for you to have a significant impact on the life of the person sitting in your office or lying in the hospital bed.

Also, this seems to be a reasonable time to address the presence of others in the room. I have definitely learned to ask, "And who do we have here?"

Presuming that someone is a parent, wife, husband, daughter, sister, friend, or other companion can definitely leave you navigating a very awkward scenario after gesturing to the patient's wife and saying, "And this must be your lovely daughter!"

## *Embracing Authenticity in Patient Interaction*

Now, to be fair, I must acknowledge that I did not first start my clinical practice or training with the level of comfort that I have recently come into. As I get to know myself and the art of medicine more intimately, I have come to appreciate more and more that patients are just people, that they have personalities, just like you do, and that connecting with them is important and appreciated.

I began to become more comfortable just being me, and I must say, the response and feedback have been astounding. Patients enjoy getting to know the real you. A patient of mine recently referred to our follow-up visit as a 'get together'. I guess I should take that to mean that they felt quite comfortable.

## *Practical Aspects of Patient Acknowledgment*

As a physician, calling the patient's name as you introduce yourself also serves a more practical purpose. It ensures that you are in the right room, with the right patient, at the right time, for the right reason.

Anyone who has spent any time in a hospital knows that it's not that difficult to walk into a patient's room and start talking to someone only to find out that you have entered the wrong room or have approached the wrong bed and started talking to the wrong patient about the wrong condition or procedure.

This is certainly awkward to navigate, and as a matter of style, I would simply apologize for the error and advise the patient that it was a pleasure meeting them nonetheless and state that it is probably good that they do not require my services at this time. I would wish them well and exit the space.

## *'Time Out' for Accuracy and Reflection*

Not only is this a humbling and scary position to be in, but this can lead to significant medical errors, and has!

To the best of my knowledge, the idea of formalizing and naming the actual process of the identification of the correct patient, procedure, and site was introduced in 2003 by the Joint Commission in the form of a 'Time Out'[1].

During a 'Time Out', we pause and verify with the patient and other team members that we are about to perform the correct intervention, on the correct patient, at the right time, on the right site, and this is a formal procedure that is also documented and verified by more than one person before proceeding.

This is so important. Could you imagine performing surgery on the wrong patient or performing a knee replacement on the wrong knee? It CAN happen, so the power of acknowledgment is of profound importance on many levels.

I love the idea of a 'Time Out', to step back and (literally) 'take a look' before acting. I believe that it has so many practical implications in the practice of medicine and any other undertaking in life that can have lasting or powerful outcomes.

A 'time out' can even serve as a call to self-reflection. What am I doing right now? Is this the right thing for me? Is this the right time for me to be doing this? Am I approaching this appropriately? If not, then think again!

So, once again, in connecting with a patient, not only are you making a good and necessary medical decision by confirming with whom you are speaking, but you are connecting with your patient and acknowledging both your and their humanity when you address them by their name.

## *Humanizing Patient Care Beyond Diagnosis*

This need to call a patient by their name seems so obvious, but it's not. Confirmation of the patient's identity is so important.

In medicine, often on ward rounds, you could hear a member of the team referring to a bed number and a diagnosis and proceeding with the plan of action for the day. Such a dehumanizing and heart-wrenching experience to watch a patient sit there and accept being identified as a diagnosis or a stage or disease or a symptom.

I remember one time after doing my early morning rounds as a junior member of a team, walking into the room and getting to know the patient before the rest of the team came so that I could present her 'case'.

This was the usual duty of the juniors. I will never forget watching one of the most senior members of the team, after talking about the 'pneumonia in bed 3' reaching to open the patient's gown from the back to listen to her lungs and subsequently being told 'Oh no!!... you will not examine me!... she (pointing at me) can examine me ...but you will not touch me!'

This was a powerful moment and I wanted to cry because I was so happy to see this person 'stand up' and demand to be treated as a person and not as a diagnosis. She refused to be touched by the senior physician who described her as a diagnosis after entering the room, without even an introduction or attempt to acknowledge her existence as anything other than a pneumonia, or ask her permission to be 'publicly' examined.

She was a person being treated for pneumonia! She was NOT a PNEUMONIA in BED 3!! But these habits are so easily passed on and perpetuated to those behind us.

Imagine walking into the ward to visit your mom or another relative or friend, only to hear the medical team talking about the UTI in room 4, the prostate cancer in room 208, or the heart failure in the ICU.

Yes, there is an absolute need for the protection of medical health information and therefore the need for confidentiality and anonymity goes without saying. But it doesn't take MUCH longer to say 'the lady in bed 3 with pneumonia' than it does to say 'the pneumonia in bed 3', but it makes such a potent statement about how you regard that person. It acknowledges to the members of the team and the staff that you regard your patient as a person and not a diagnosis.

I believe that the lady was angry because she sat and listened as this doctor came in with the team and started talking about the pneumonia in the bed. She was probably livid that this doctor would walk up to her and attempt to open the back of her gown without so much as an acknowledgment.

We sometimes forget that our patients are people, intelligent people, people with jobs and lives and families and all the things that we have.

Remember that your patient is a woman with pneumonia or a lady with cervical cancer, she is not a pneumonia or a cervical cancer! Be careful how you refer to patients in private; it may come out of your mouth in public.

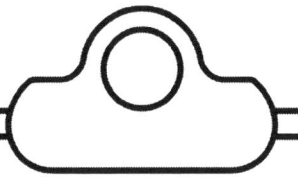

## BOTTOM LINE

Acknowledge that your patient is a person.

Address them as such.

Address them as you would want to be addressed if you were a patient. You might just be one day!!

# ℞ ACTION PLAN

- [ ] Reflect on ways that you could implement each of the suggestions into your practice in a meaningful way.

- [ ] Think of times when you may not have done so.

## Chapter 3

# The Power of Courtesy

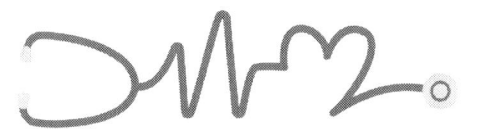

So, as I thought about the angle I would take when approaching this topic, I was kind of blindsided by what came to me. What we are going to talk about here is being courteous to your patient. I know, right!? Again, I am sure you won't anticipate where I am going with this...but here goes nothing.

### *The Importance of Being on Time*

Picture this: you are the surgical oncology fellow at one of the most prestigious hospitals in the country, and you are on for the afternoon clinic. The resident (specialist doctor in training) has been there taking histories and doing exams but can't 'dispo' (discharge or dismiss) the patient until you or the attending (Consultant) arrives.

The surgery case you were in this morning was really complicated as the vascularity was significantly more than anyone had anticipated, so you are 2 hours late for the clinic.

So, you swoop into the clinic, enter the first exam room, and listen to the H&P. The resident says to the patient, 'This is Dr. Brown,' and you briefly nod in acknowledgment, examine the patient, tell the resident what to do, and then move onto the next room with the next resident. You manage to clear the clinic over the next two hours and leave for home completely exhausted to get some well-deserved rest.

Fast forward to 8 years later, when that surgical resident finished his residency and fellowship in surgical oncology, finally landed his dream job, and joined a very successful and well-reputed group practice.

Ten months into his new position, he had a meeting with the practice manager because he has an unusually high no-show rate for follow-ups and a declining number of encounters that translate into actual surgical procedures.

He has a great reputation for first-time consultations because of the accolades with which he graduated, the institution from which he graduated, and because of his plethora of publications and association memberships. His bio on the practice website is glowing and quite impeccable, and he knows it.

So, what was happening? He and his practice manager had several meetings thereafter to try to find the source of the problem. His surgical complication rate was low, but the percentage of patient encounters that led to him being the primary surgeon was lower compared to other members of the group.

What was the problem? He was often late for appointments and rarely apologized, barely introduced himself to patients, and made little effort to make them feel comfortable.

I suppose he took for granted the fact that he was a great surgeon and figured that if patients wanted to see him, then they would wait for him and be grateful that he showed up to take care of them.

He figured that if they made an appointment to see him, then they obviously knew who he was and how good he was at performing surgery, which he certainly was.

I guess he believed that his 'CV' spoke for itself and that his qualifications would automatically lead to a thriving practice. Think back to his experience as a resident; the fellow (senior specialist in training) rarely acknowledged the patients and was focused only on hearing the story and getting the clinic emptied so that he could go home.

## *Acknowledging Your Patients*

In my practice, I sometimes fall behind on appointment times. I try not to double-book appointments although we all know why practices do this sometimes. Often patients don't show up for appointments, so sometimes we may double book a few spots in case someone does not show up.

Depending on how busy the practice is, there is sometimes a long wait to get an appointment, and so it feels like a complete waste when patients 'no show' for an appointment, even after confirming, especially when someone else has been put on a waiting list for the same spot.

Sometimes a patient waits several weeks for another spot when they could have had the time slot allotted to someone who 'no showed'. Patients seem not to understand this, or care, I guess.

But still, I make it a practice not to routinely double-book my appointments. I also try to be respectful of the patient's time. I suppose a compromise can be to shorten the appointment slots, and this allows more time for an encounter if people don't show up. It also allows you to cut down on the wait time to get an appointment.

## *The Value of Apologizing*

I always apologize when I am late for a patient encounter. Sometimes, I explain what happened and sometimes I don't, but I always take the time to acknowledge to the patient that I believe that their time is important and valuable and that sometimes in my field, unexpected things happen that cause me to run behind.

I apologize! I really do feel that the time of the patient is valuable, and I genuinely mean it when I apologize.

I can't tell you how many times a patient has been in the waiting room 'raising hell' with the staff about the time that they have been waiting (which is rarely more than about 30 minutes... but that's another story), who leave the encounter laughing and completely satisfied.

In addition, you can see the body language of a patient change completely when you walk into the office and apologize, if only briefly, for keeping them waiting. Everyone wants to be viewed as valuable.

No one wants to feel taken for granted, and let's face it, if you didn't have patients, then you wouldn't be much of a doctor. So, the value of the apology is not really taught in formal medical training, not in my experience. But it can easily bridge the gap between a resentful and dissatisfied patient and a grateful one.

## *Managing Patient Expectations*

Confession time. So, I really do appreciate the apology, because even though as a doctor, I completely understand, in theory, what causes patients to have to wait, I am a completely irrational patient lol. I hate waiting.

I don't understand why, if my appointment is at 1 PM, I cannot be in the room by 1:15 or at least 1:30. Truthfully, I want to be in at '1 on the dot' lol...unless I'm late, in which case I want to walk right in because I gave you extra time to catch up.

As a physician, I know what's happening in the back there and I still get a little impatient sometimes, which is completely ridiculous, but may explain why I am so empathetic when it comes to tardiness in my clinic.

And I certainly do hold a grudge when I am kept waiting for a ridiculous amount of time by a doctor and receive no apology or acknowledgment. Just say sorry. It's not a sign of weakness. It's just plain polite.

## Reflecting on Patient Wait Times

Truthfully, I witnessed something in a waiting room once that totally enlightened me. It changed me a little and made me even more likely to apologize to a patient. I was in a waiting room when I witnessed a patient go up to the receptionist counter.

The patient politely (albeit loudly) advised the waiting room staff that he was a professional who billed by the hour and that his bill per hour was far more than the doctor's bill. He advised the staff that his office was nearby and that they should call him when the doctor was nearly ready, or he would send the doctor a bill for the hours he spent waiting for him.

Now truthfully, this was a bit extreme of an example, but it happened. The patient had been waiting for nearly four hours, which is also an extreme amount of time, but he was right!

We often think of our time as more valuable than that of the people that we serve. We implicitly believe that they should wait any amount of time that it takes.

Some attorneys, business execs, and other professionals do bill more per hour than we could ever dream of billing; and yes, the service that we provide is sometimes needed for their actual survival, but that does not mean that we should take them for granted.

We should treat each of our patients as important, and imagine if we were stuck in the waiting room with our child or parent waiting for 3 hours for an appointment.

## Respecting Patient Time

I live and work in a small community and sometimes patients would come for their appointments during their lunch hour. They are employed and must clock in and out of their places of work.

So, you can see how in this scenario, sitting in the waiting room for 40 minutes to see the doctor is impractical. How could they see me and have a meaningful appointment and drive back to work which is 20 minutes away with only 20 minutes left before they must clock back in?

Furthermore, clinic hours are often regular office business hours, and not everyone can take a day off to see the doctor. So, you see, for patients managing chronic medical conditions, where regular follow-up is necessary, the convenience of the appointment is going to affect how reliable a patient is at keeping their follow-up visits.

Honestly, for those who work nearby, I tell them to call my staff a little before their appointment time and liaise with the staff about how it's going so that they can time themselves, and while this may not always be feasible, it helps to bring awareness to you as you take care of your patients.

Remember that they are people; working, living people, with schedules sometimes just as hectic as yours. Be compassionate.

## *Establishing Mutual Respect*

Now, this is not at all to suggest that you are a complete pushover!! There must be balance and mutual respect established in these relationships. In the practice of medicine, we accept that exceptional situations will arise and that no matter how much we plan, someone will always blindside us with a 'doorknob' confession that makes every sphincter in your entire body contract.

You stare at the patient and think to yourself, we just spent 20 minutes together. Why would you tell me this as I am leaving the room to go to the next patient? I'll take this a step further.

We have all been the resident rotating in the ER at the end of the shift who thinks, 'You have had this headache for the past 12 weeks. Why did you choose tonight, at the end of my shift, to show up?' lol. Some of us have even asked the patient, partially as a part of history taking and partially as an act of passive aggression, 'What made you come in TONIGHT???!!!'

Well, back to my office where my diabetic patient now casually decides to tell me about this discomfort in her chest that happens only sometimes and doesn't last very long. This is that 5 seconds where you decide, do I get into this now, or can this be dealt with at the next visit?

Well, when it comes to the diabetic woman in her late 40s or 50s who has atypical chest discomfort, this is probably not an issue that we should tackle at the next visit. We need to unpack this now.

And yes, it has been happening for months, and no, she has not mentioned it to anyone else, and yes, she has seen several doctors during that time, and no…she did not mention it to any of them, and yes… she did her annual physical last week and said nothing…and yes she chose to mention it to you!

Fast forward 10 minutes later after you have taken your chest pain history, just like they taught you in medical school, you pick up the phone and call the cardiologist's office and make her appointment, and she is seeing him tomorrow or next week…you can't quite recall…but it's an expedited visit.

It's a good thing you called because when you see her a few weeks later, she is status post stress test and cardiac catheterization and stent placement!!! And yes, she came to see you about a thyroid nodule, not for diabetes and certainly not for chest pain.

So, now you are a full 20-30 minutes behind and you walk into the room of the next patient who has been waiting for some time, but not an unreasonable amount of time. You have been busting your tail and you are tired and exhausted, and you are doing far more than you bargained for that day because you have been taking time to field your patient concerns to this point.

Before the patient with the chest pain, there was another patient who showed up unannounced and without an appointment, because she claimed that she could not get through to the office. She felt so bad that she decided to show up because she felt that she would either die or end up in the emergency room if she didn't see you because she felt so badly. And it's a good thing she did show up because she was remarkably thyrotoxic with a heart rate of 120 beats per minute and was severely symptomatic. Never mind the fact that she discontinued her medication to see what would happen.

So, you put out that fire, and as you enter the room of the next scheduled patient, he looks at you enraged and goes on with his derogatory remarks about how he does not know why doctors schedule more patients than they can see. He carried on with his condescending discourse about how if I wanted to keep him as a patient, then I needed to figure out how to be on time, and he advised me that he was about to walk out and that I had 5 minutes to see him and that I'd better hurry up. True story!

Needless to say, even I, 'sister Mary-cheerful' as I had been once addressed, was NOT A HAPPY CAMPER. I took a very visibly deep breath. I looked at him squarely and I smiled briefly (yes, I did smile). I said something like this; 'Sir, I am sincerely sorry for your wait, and I do respect your time and I do not typically overbook my schedule, but you must understand that I am a doctor, and sometimes people will walk into my office and say things that completely throw me off course.

Someone may walk in with a blood pressure of 200/102, a heart rate of 120 bpm, or chest pain that was not on the list of things that I planned to address that day. This means that sometimes I will have to help a patient navigate an emergency that can cause my schedule to run off course.

One day that patient might be you. I have specialized knowledge that may be of benefit to you and the management of your condition, and if you believe that these interactions, inclusive of the possible unplanned wait times, are not worth it for you, you can feel free to see someone else.

Only you can make that decision. I can't do that for you. Now, would you like to proceed with this appointment?' Without a smile, he gestured for me to sit, and we continued with a very interesting visit.

Of course, the next time I saw his name on my schedule, I swore that he would not show up, but I tried to hurry along so as to minimize the wait time for him if he did indeed decide to come.

Of course, I fell behind and as I entered the room a few minutes after the appointment time, I smiled and said, "Hello sir, I'm sorry for the wait!"

He looked at me as if I had a frog on my nose and said, "Why are you apologizing to me?" I was dumbfounded. What I hadn't mentioned was how this man walked out of my exam room and left the office on more than one occasion because, as far as he was concerned, I had him waiting too long.

This was before the encounter referenced above. So, I was not expecting this response from him. But I carried on with the visit and on every subsequent visit, even if there was a wait, I would apologize and carry on and he never spoke of our encounter again.

What am I saying? You can be courteous and also demand the respect that you deserve for your sacrifice, all at the same time. I am by no means saying that by being courteous and respectful of patients, you should allow yourself to be bullied or 'run over' by someone who refuses to consider your point of view in it all.

Sometimes they need to be brought up to speed about the nuances of clinical practice. And you will lose some patients because of it, but not the patients that really want to benefit from your knowledge and experience. It is beyond the scope of this current writing to discuss the effect of wait times on patient satisfaction scores as a measure of the quality of a patient experience at a healthcare facility, nor is it my intention to discuss this issue.

But suffice it to say, that when prolonged wait times are necessary, it's probably better when there is a genuine, but brief apology involved, as opposed to completely failing to acknowledge that the inconvenience has occurred. For many of us in a hired physician model, patient satisfaction is a measure that can come up at evaluations. So, this is just a brief citing of that fact.

## *Effective Coping Mechanisms*

Another aspect of acknowledging yourself as human and vulnerable is to recognize that stressful scenarios require effective coping mechanisms. It is important to figure out little or big things that you can do to manage this pressure in a reasonable way.

I remember one of my medical assistants asking me one day, "Dr. Parker, how do you manage to be happy for the entire day and why do we never see you angry?" I openly and honestly told her that when I got frustrated and overwhelmed, I would go to the restroom or into my office, close the door, and let it out.

Honestly, sometimes I would stare out of the window for 3 minutes and think of nothing, or people watch, or crack a joke to myself and then regroup. Sometimes I pray. Sometimes I try to muffle a scream and honestly, I have even cried during the early years of training. Sometimes I check text messages or send messages or read silly memes and laugh out loud, I may open my junk mail from my favorite stores, or I may add something to my shopping cart if it is on my mind, even if I never purchase it, anything to disconnect for a moment from the stress.

Once I have reset, which generally takes about 1 minute or 2-3 if it's bad, then I can get on with the day. Another tactic is that when annoying calls come, I will let out how I really feel before I pick up the phone so that by the time I pick up the phone I can be genuinely nice and receptive because I have already gotten over the burden of the extra work that it will engender.

Another way to help manage the load is to learn to delegate tasks to others that you can train and trust to do them well. This was very hard for me to do but was so necessary and helpful.

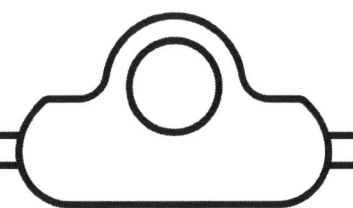

## BOTTOM LINE

Your patient's time is valuable and so is yours.

Be courteous to your patients, but also demand that they respect you as you do them.

Acknowledge to your patient that waiting is annoying, but that sometimes it is necessary and is generally not the intended outcome.

Your job is stressful, and you need to develop healthy and effective ways to manage this.

You may need to talk to a professional if you are not finding effective ways to manage your stress.

# ℞ ACTION PLAN

- [ ] Apologize for being a little late the next time you keep a patient waiting and watch the surprise on their face if you have never done so before.

- [ ] Remember it doesn't have to be a production, a simple 'sorry for the wait' will do.

- [ ] Think of a quick pep-talk or action that you can take throughout the day, privately or not, that can help you to release steam so as to not become overburdened by the work of the day. Find ways to inject pleasure or stress relievers into your day.

- [ ] Seek help if you need it.

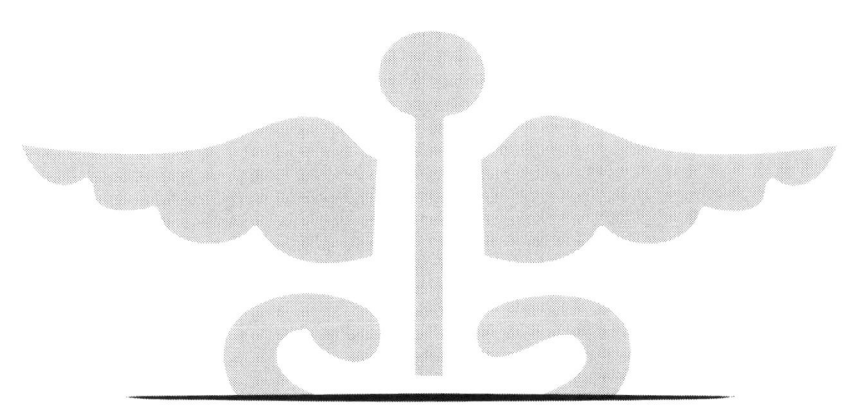

# SECTION 2
# AWARENESS

# AWARENESS

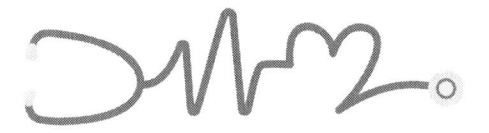

"As you RACE through your Day, Don't Forget to C.A.R.E."

## "A" is for AWARENESS

The power steps we'll explore in this section highlight the importance of being conscious of your surroundings, your patients, their expressions, your own expressions, and the presence of others in the room.

Being mindful of yourself and how your actions affect others and influence interactions can significantly enhance your ability to manage encounters. Our habits, tendencies, behaviors, postures, and positions profoundly impact patient encounters. This makes it crucial to become aware of how what we do and how we do it shapes our relationships with others.

I understand that maintaining this awareness can be challenging, especially for busy residents and hospitalists who are often exhausted and eager to complete tasks as swiftly as possible.

This urgency can lead to closed postures and other nonverbal cues signaling to the patient the need for brevity. Sometimes, this message is conveyed more directly. However, I recommend taking a deep breath before entering the room and striving to remain composed, even under time constraints.

Let's discuss how increased awareness can positively influence our day-to-day interactions.

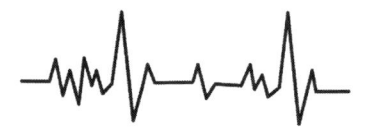

## Chapter 4

# The Power of Your Physical Positioning in the Room

When I enter a patient room, which for me is typically in the outpatient setting, I try to establish myself as accessible and relatable as soon as possible.

Initially, this may have developed because it was more comfortable for me, but ultimately, I noticed that it was more comfortable for the patient. If I enter a room in which a patient is already seated, I would quickly greet them and take my seat in the chair.

*Tailoring Your Approach to Clinical Settings*

During very brief follow-up visits, it can be tempting and sometimes even appropriate for you to remain standing as the patient sits. These recommendations must be tailored to the clinical setting and not applied in a blanket fashion.

For instance, if you are running the suture removal clinic, you may well just introduce yourself, and review the mode of injury and the date of suture placement. The patient may already have been 'prepped' by the nurse or assistant and is simply awaiting your arrival. A long drawn-out conversation might actually be weird in this setting. Get in, assess the patient, remove the sutures, and 'dispo' the patient with follow-up as appropriate.

## *Building Rapport in Clinical Practice*

Now, in the clinical setting where you are building rapport with patients that you seek to retain in your practice, then your investment in relationship building is well worth the effort. Remaining standing, especially if a patient and his or her family member is seated in a chair, placing them significantly below your eye level for the encounter, can create a physical barrier to your connection. A patient seated on the exam table probably eliminates this differential, depending on your height.

I find that speaking down to a patient for a long period of time can be intimidating and just uncomfortable because the patient must exert such great effort to maintain an upward gaze. Sitting next to the patient at eye level, if only for a moment, can communicate a degree of accessibility to you and what you have to offer.

## *The Importance of Sitting Down with Patients*

This is also true in the hospital setting. This obviously will be dependent on many factors. If you have a busy team of 23 patients to round on this morning because you accepted night float, and you have a resident and two interns, a sub-intern, and a medical student on your team, and you have to get to noon conference and teach the students after rounds; then sitting on the chair next to every patient is clearly not practical.

But there may be one or two instances where the extra 2 minutes on rounds could have a significant impact on your patient, on you, and on the student and young doctors that you are coaching with your words and actions.

A young college student, a non-smoker, on his way to grad school who presented to the hospital because of a chronic intermittent cough, is now grappling with a new diagnosis of lung cancer. This patient had hopes and dreams that he may never get to fulfill. A few minutes to sit on the visitor's chair and let him know that the team will do all that they can to help him may go a long way to helping his morale and bolstering the 'fight' in him that he may need to face the road ahead.

We never truly know the inner pinings, secrets, and situations that patients struggle with, and it can be so easy to consider patients as diagnoses, but when these things hit very close to home, they can change you. Always remember that this patient may be 'just' a patient to you, but when it's someone close to you, they are never JUST a patient!

## *A Personal Anecdote: Understanding Patients Beyond Diagnoses*

I remember being the junior member of the medical team and I was doing my pre-rounds so that I could present my patient to the seniors before ward rounds. I can vividly remember what happened one morning at around 7 AM. I was sitting in the chair next to the patient asking her how she was doing. I can't actually remember why she was admitted to our team, but I remember her telling me that she wanted to tell me something. So, I told her that she could go ahead.

She began to tell me the story about how a few weeks ago she had fallen in the tub and had gotten a bruise on her left breast. She was nursing the bruise initially with some ice packs and eventually with some creams and salves, but she was concerned because it was getting worse. She told me that it wasn't hurting anymore but that the swelling had not gone down yet so she was a bit concerned.

She figured that since she was in the hospital, she should mention it to someone. So, I asked her if she would like me to take a look at it and she said that she was scared but she agreed to the exam. I told her that I would look at the normal breast first just to be sure and then she permitted me to examine the left breast.

When she removed the gown on the left, what I saw changed me forever, but I smiled at her and told her that I would just feel it to check. With my gloved hand, I examined her left breast and axilla, and it felt like a bag of concrete and there were little pebbles under the armpit also. The skin was stuck to the breast and the breast was kind of stuck to the chest wall.

There were no ulcerations in the skin or discharge from the nipple, but the skin was abnormally thick and pitted like the peel of an orange. Clearly, this was not the result of a slip and fall in the tub a few weeks prior. What this was...was a cry for help. She was clearly petrified but decided that she had found someone that she could share this with. She begged me not to tell her sister or anyone who visited her.

Obviously, I agreed, but I advised her that I would have to tell my seniors so that the appropriate specialist consultations and management could be initiated for her. She agreed to this, and I left the room holding back tears. She must have been in denial for months.

## *Key Strategies for Connecting with Patients*

When establishing rapport with the patient by paying attention to body language, establishing the appropriate amount of eye contact, and interacting with your patient with appropriate communicative touches; you will find that this is all more easily facilitated when you are at eye level with the patient.

Connecting with a patient can prompt them to give information that they have been withholding from anyone else, and sometimes this information is riveting.

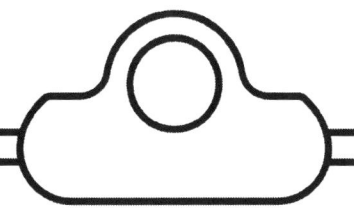

## BOTTOM LINE

Standing over a patient for a prolonged period can be uncomfortable for a patient, even if they are lying in a hospital bed. Sitting on the chair, if only for 30 seconds to place your hand on the bed briefly (or better yet on the patient's shoulder as appropriate), while you summarize the plan, can speak volumes to your humanity. This can make the patient feel cared for and not just admitted to your service.

When a patient feels cared for, they appreciate it.

When a patient feels cared for, they will entrust you with information that can help you to help them.

# ℞ ACTION PLAN

- [ ] Once or twice in your day, try to sit next to a patient for the interaction, in part or in whole. This is of course relevant for those of us who do not typically sit during patient encounters.

# Chapter 5

# The Power of Listening

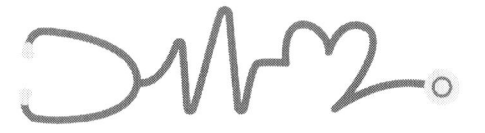

So, you've introduced yourself and you have asked the patient what has brought them there to see you today. Are you ready to listen to the answer? In the practice of medicine and in the practice of life, we are constantly in a time crunch.

We are always living in the next moment because we have 20 patients to see in the clinic or we must finish rounds and hurry off to the office, or we have to hurry up because we have to catch a lecture.

We have administrators telling us how much time we are allowed to spend with each patient and sometimes these administrators have no clinical experience.

The art of medicine is also being challenged by the burden of documentation and the need to satisfy someone's idea of quality measures that are now built into an electronic medical record.

Sometimes you cannot even progress to the next step in your documentation process before checking a mandatory box or progressing through an administrative roadblock from which you cannot reverse or divert.

I am certainly not suggesting that these things do not have their (proven) merit, or that they are not useful and even necessary in some instances. I am simply saying that they are increasing the demands placed on the already burdened physician.

The more we progress in medicine, the more challenging it is to practice and the more pressure there is with competing non-clinical obligations. Doctoring is tough.

Many consider pivoting to careers in other fields simply because of the ever-increasing demands that go along with the practice of medicine.

## *The Challenge of Time Management*

We must still somehow find the time to listen to what the patient is saying. In general, studies are showing that physicians allow patients less than 10-12 seconds of free speaking before the first interruption occurs.[1]

Now, the estimate of the amount of time before the first interruption varies slightly depending on the source of the information, but the bottom line remains the same, it's NOT a very long time. The interruptions occur for many different reasons, but nonetheless serve as an impediment to the most effective communication.

## *Strategies for Effective Communication*

In my lectures, I often advise physicians who have long-term patients with multiple chronic medical illnesses to set goals for each clinical encounter.

This allows the patient to express what they feel is most important to be addressed in that visit, and also allows you to make sure that you are also addressing what is most important for you to accomplish during that encounter after making sure that the patient is overall medically 'stable'.

For instance, in managing the diabetic patient, I have a (mental) checklist and after about 2 to 3 encounters, we would have completed all the things on the checklist.

Initially, your checklist might need to be a physical one that you keep handy.

At the end of each visit, I would make a quick note of what we addressed and of the things that need to be addressed at the subsequent visits.

This allows for some 'free' time to discuss patient concerns in the encounters and allows the physician to set attainable goals for each encounter thereby minimizing frustration and a feeling that you are not accomplishing what is needed for the patient.

Sometimes we address two matters and table the others for future encounters.

Each item on the checklist for a patient living with diabetes who is establishing care with me would be addressed, but the order may differ depending on what is actively concerning to the patient, concerning to myself, or what may be causing complications.

Specifically, a checklist for my diabetic patient may look like this:

- Check basic labs (A1C, CBC, lipids, urine microalbumin creatinine: ratio, metabolic panel (creatinine and eGFR)).

- Review medication appropriateness and adjust as needed.

- Monofilament, pulse, skin of feet exam, and referral to podiatry if necessary

- Eye exam or referral to ophthalmology

- Make sure that age-appropriate annual screening is done and refer to a primary physician for this purpose if you are not that physician.

## *Implementing a Patient-Centered Approach*

At the end of an introductory encounter, after listening to the patient's major concerns and taking a history, I order my labs to be reviewed at the next visit.

In the absence of major concerns on vital signs or general exam that need immediate attention, I would review the patient medication list and make adjustments as appropriate, and that may be all that we do that day.

I would document that labs were ordered and that a monofilament exam, eye exam, and age-appropriate screening will be addressed at upcoming visits. By the end of the third visit, all of this would have been done.

Sometimes it all gets done in the first visit, but it depends on the complexity of the patient. Trying to do too much in the encounter can lead to everything being done poorly and/or to the patient feeling rushed.

The above scenario allows you to free up some time to listen to the patient because you have given yourself permission to pick up where you left off once you have made sure that the patient is not in need of any immediate intervention.

This paradigm does not work for every type of patient encounter, but it may be modified depending on your specialty and practice situation as appropriate.

The spare time that you have left behind might give you a moment to follow up on a tiny personal detail that reassures your patient, that to you, they are more than just a number.

A patient who feels rushed may walk away from the clinical encounter feeling 'un-listened-to' and dissatisfied and may walk away with a concern that might have been deemed urgent, should you have had the time to hear it.

Allowing yourself time to listen to the patient allows the time to make personal connections, that are small, but so powerful.

Consider, if at the last visit, the patient told you that they had to follow up in 5 weeks instead of the four weeks that you suggested, because they had to travel. At some point during the current visit, you might ask the patient, "So, did you make it over to Philadelphia after all? How was the trip?"

The patient stops and looks at you with their jaw touching the ground. "You remembered, Doc??!!! Wow. Thank you. My trip was great. We saw the Liberty Bell and did so many things." The patient says to themselves, or perhaps to you, "You are now my favorite doctor!!!"

Congratulations! Just remember, if the patient tells you something, make a tiny note of it. Mention it next time. There is something to a personal touch that simply can't be adequately described and certainly cannot be replaced or imitated.

Be a person in your patient encounter! These tools were simply things that I did naturally. I like to talk and laugh.

Most people who know me on a personal level will attest to this fact. But as I analyzed the qualities that would cause a patient to choose to see me, to choose to return to me for continued care, or choose to send their family and friends to see me, I had to take stock of the things that I did (and did not do) as a physician.

I had to consider things that I desired but didn't necessarily experience in my role as a patient and I also had to think about the things that the patients directly said were the reason that they would choose to engage me as a physician on a recurring basis. I have even had some patients say to me, "Doc, please don't change!"

This naturally led me to ponder the documentation burden I mentioned earlier. Balancing clinical excellence with administrative duties is a continuous struggle, especially since I spend considerable time interacting with patients and must remember to document during encounters.

The old adage from my training days, "If it wasn't written down, it wasn't done," resonates more profoundly now than ever.

Initially, I viewed it primarily as a medico-legal statement and as a reminder of the need to document for continuity of care and better patient management. However, as a practicing physician, I've learned that documentation is intricately tied to billing and reimbursement, adding another layer of complexity and importance to this task.

Developing clinical acumen and bedside manner must, therefore, be balanced with the need for thorough and timely documentation. Budgeting time for documentation at the end of each encounter; day; or week is crucial. That administrative day or half day becomes invaluable.

The power of listening must not overshadow the need for appropriate documentation of the relevant parts of these enriching interactions with your patients.

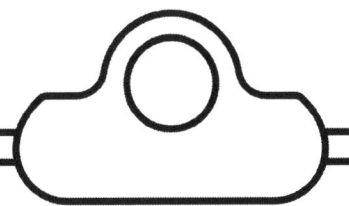

## BOTTOM LINE

Listen to the patient, including little things that they tell you about themselves that are not clinical, but that are personal. They are sharing their lives with you. It's an opportunity to connect.

Show the patient that you are listening to what they are saying by referring to things that they may have told you at previous encounters. Don't spend too much time on it as your time is limited, but spend just enough time to make it meaningful. The patient will remember this.

# ℞ ACTION PLAN

- [ ] Write things down that were significant to the patient to remind you to bring it up briefly at the follow up visit.

- [ ] Remember that in some practice settings, it is ok to address other issues at a further visit, even if you have to schedule a visit sooner than usual to make sure that all concerns are covered.

# The Power of Listening

## PART 2: THE DIAGNOSTIC VALUE OF LISTENING

There is another more clinical aspect of listening to a patient that we need to discuss.

Let's talk about this here. I remember being taught somewhere along the way that about 80-90% of the diagnosis is in the history and the physical exam, and that ancillary tests are confirmatory tools. I have a few stories about how this can be relevant.

We have already discussed our tendency to interrupt the patient for many reasons, and we have quantified just how quick we are to interrupt. Interruptions, although sometimes necessary, can take many forms.

Perhaps the cellphone rings, sometimes the pager goes off, sometimes the patient is veering off course with a story or unrelated concern, sometimes you really are pressed for time and would prefer a more problem-focused approach for this encounter.

Sometimes the patient really is talking a lot, and sometimes you have had a long day and a longer week. But sometimes, just sometimes, you think you know what the patient is about to tell you or is trying to tell you, so you jump in with the proverbial "I got you".

Because of your brilliance, experience, medical knowledge, intuition, and ability to recognize clinical signs and symptoms in patients, you will be correct…MUCH of the time; probably even most of the time. But, be very wary of this.

## *A Lesson from the Emergency Room*

I remember a story about an experience that an intern once had. It may even have been a medical student, but let's go with intern for the purposes of this telling.

There was a patient in the ER (Emergency Room) who had advised the intern interviewing him that he was having difficulty breathing. The patient apparently reported that he felt like something was squeezing his neck and that he couldn't breathe.

He felt like someone was standing and squeezing him around the neck from the outside. It was difficult for him to describe exactly when he started to feel this way, but certainly, it began to worsen significantly enough for him to seek emergency medical attention.

After the patient gave the history of his complaint, his 'case' was presented to the attending physician (consultant doctor or doctor in charge). The intern intended to have the patient presented to the Internal Medicine service for admission and management of an asthma attack.

The reviewing attending was astonished about this proposed asthma admission, where there was no mention of wheezing, shortness of breath, tightness in the chest, or even a personal or family history of asthma.

'Why am I admitting this patient to the medical service?' the attending asked the intern. 'For asthma' was the response. The attending doctor said 'Seriously?!' and rolled his eyes. 'This does not sound like an asthma attack to me!

'This patient is telling you that something is squeezing his throat and you are not listening to him. I cannot present this patient to the medical service, and I'm not releasing him from the ER until you assess the patient for what he is complaining about.'

'He does not likely have asthma' the attending said, 'and if there is not someone visible to you standing in the room squeezing this patient's neck from the outside, then I suggest that you examine him again and get a 'CAT scan' of the neck!'

The intern was taken aback but definitely began to rethink how confident she was with her 'bread and butter' diagnosis. She was convinced that the brief history that she took and the 'focused' physical examination that she performed had led her directly to his obvious diagnosis of asthma.

The attending went on to say 'This sounds like an upper airway issue', and she proceeded to accompany the intern to the bedside of the patient and asked the intern to take a brief history of the patient's complaint and to examine the patient quickly while she remained in the room to assess the patient with her.

Ultimately, the 'CAT scan' of the neck was completed, and the attending took the intern with her to the radiology reading room immediately to have the images reviewed by the resident radiologist on call.

After a brief review of the images showing deviation of the trachea and a significant degree of compression, ENT (The Ear Nose & Throat Specialist) was called to the ER to assess the patient for an emergency controlled intubation for tracheal deviation and impending airway obstruction.

The patient was taken to the OR (operating room) in case the intubation failed and warranted an emergency tracheostomy (surgical airway).

Needless to say, the intern learned a very important lesson that day, which of course is the whole point of an internship. The patient had described quite precisely what was happening to him. His airway was being compressed by something external to it.

Perhaps he had a large goiter. But we will never know...what we do know is that listening carefully to this patient's story prevented him from having an acutely obstructed airway (a surgical/ENT emergency) while being managed on the medical service for the asthma, which he did not have. If this patient was indeed admitted to the medical service, it could have led to a catastrophe.

## *Key Takeaways*

So, the lessons here are many, but we will address two of them. First, the intern doctor heard the patient, took a great history, and documented exactly what the patient told her.

But, never once did she actually listen to the patient. The patient told her exactly what was going on. There was an obstruction in his upper airway. That's what he told her, not quite in those words, but that's precisely what he described to her.

So, I'm not certain if it was that she decided that the patient had asthma, if she was tired, if she didn't feel like listening so she 'slapped a diagnosis' on the chart, or if her experience to that point, was simply not leading her to think of something outside of asthma, or if it was that she didn't feel that the patient was capable of giving an intelligent description of what he was experiencing (we can be very judgmental at times).

Perhaps there was a little of each of the above contributing to what went on. Perhaps there was more. Perhaps the intern doctor simply didn't make the connection between the patient's description of what was happening to him and what the likely differential diagnoses could have been. Perhaps, she genuinely thought that this patient had asthma. This was probably the case.

The bottom line here is to try to listen to the patient as this will likely help to guide you to the appropriate explanation for the patient's symptoms; and as your experience and clinical acumen matures, your list of differentials will become more exhaustive and precise at the same time.

The second area of this scenario that needs attention is the clinical acumen of the attending physician to surmise the likely scenario from the history that the intern took. The intern did in fact take an awesome history. The attending listened to the history and immediately picked up that the story that the patient told and the diagnosis that the intern doctor gave were incongruent.

Had she not listened to her intern describe the complaint that the patient had, she would have missed that this diagnosis simply didn't make sense. Clearly, the patient would have been examined by the attending regardless of the intern's presentation of the case, but you get the point.

Use your ears and eyes twice as much as you use your mouth. It will pay off! You have two ears and two eyes but only ONE MOUTH!! Listen carefully and observe critically.

## *The Value of Internship in Medical Training*

This is by no means an attack on interns. We all have our stories. The whole point of internship is to gain exposure and to receive guidance from our seniors and colleagues. If we are now physicians, then we have once been interns.

Internship is the breeding ground for perfection, so take in every mistake and learn from it, lean into the experience, tired and exhausted though you may be, this too shall pass, and you will soon miss the protection afforded to those who are 'lowly' interns.

During this time of internship and residency, there is intense pressure to acquire and perfect clinical knowledge. At the same time, you must translate this into being able to actually see a patient and come up with an accurate diagnosis and a reasonable and guideline-based plan of action. You must learn to interact with patients, colleagues, and other staff members all while being sleep-deprived and overworked.

We must take time to recharge even in these moments, as at this stage, many of us are questioning our choice. I remember getting through this by telling myself that it couldn't possibly last forever. I was also able to encourage many of those that came behind me. That does not mean that I did not struggle. We all do.

The struggles are professional and personal. We are trying to balance work life, family life, lack of family life, relationships, lack of relationships, and so many other concerns that we as humans face. Yes, doctor...you are also a human, with human needs and desires and frailties.

## *Valuing Connections Beyond the Clinic*

During these moments, spending time with friends and colleagues is so important, even if you are dog-tired; because the memories that you create help to sustain you through the tougher moments.

I remember going to discount movies on Tuesday nights with my friends, some of the movies I didn't necessarily want to see, but it didn't really matter because I got out and spent time with my friends. I remember those moments even now, despite the fact that some of the friendships have faded.

We will always have those times that we spent together helping each other survive and even thrive. Please remember to try to find balance and to find small moments to steal away and recharge and consider the other things that matter to you.

If I had known then what I know now, I would have gone out even more, despite my immense fatigue.

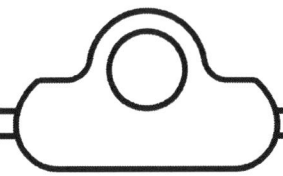

## BOTTOM LINE

Listen to your patients.

Listen to your colleagues.

Listen to yourself.

# ℞ ACTION PLAN

☐ Be intentional about listening to the patient while they are speaking. Feel free to redirect patients that are veering too far off course; but invest in actually listening, and not assuming that you know what they are going to say or are trying to say.

☐ Take care to listen to your emotions and to address them, especially when you feel vulnerable. Find a friend to hang out with sometimes.

# The Power of Listening

## *Part 3: Listening Beyond the Obvious*

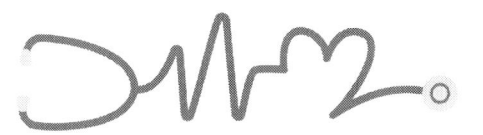

Another important point that must be emphasized now, is the importance of listening to a patient even when they walk in the door with a diagnosis. It could be wrong, or there could be more to the story than meets the eye.

Let's talk about another story that can help to illustrate the power of listening to the patient and not necessarily accepting the labels that they come with.

### *A Case of Misdiagnosed Eye Disease*

There was a patient being managed for Graves' disease who eventually decided to seek the care of an endocrinologist. He presented himself for transfer of care, and the doctor began to take a history.

They started from the beginning, with him describing when he was diagnosed with hyperthyroidism, and they went on to discuss his other medical history, allergies, family history, and all the usual questions that a doctor would ask a patient.

He went on to tell the doctor that he had Graves' eye disease. The doctor looked at him quite curiously and asked him to describe exactly what he meant. He went on to say that his doctors told him that he has Graves' disease and that therefore his eye complaints were because of Graves' eye disease.

He didn't appear to have the typical findings associated with thyroid eye disease, so the doctor asked him to describe any symptoms that he may have been experiencing.

He stated that sometimes one eye might appear to be more prominent or more open than the other, but that there was no real bulging of the eyeballs out of the socket. He denied an inability to close his eyes, the sensation of dryness of the eyes, or the sensation of grittiness in the eyes that could imply incomplete closure that can happen in thyroid eye disease.

He went on to tell the endocrinologist that what he experienced was quite the opposite. He stated that at the beginning of the day, he was great; he could see, and that his eyes were wide open and symmetrical, and that he could work well and effectively.

He stated that later in the day, it would start to feel like his eyelids were drooping and that somehow, even though he was not actually physically tired or fatigued, he physically couldn't keep his eyes open. Sometimes he would have to mechanically keep an eyelid open by using his fingers to hold the upper lids up.

This had been going on for years, and he had compensated for this and ended days early so he could drive. He said that if he rested, even if he wasn't exactly sleepy, it would reliably get better.

So, the doctor looked at him, flabbergasted, and asked him if he had told his doctors that this was what he was experiencing. He definitively said yes!! That's the Thyroid Eye Disease that they diagnosed me with.

He was hoping that it would have gotten better with the hyperthyroidism treatment over the years because they said that it likely would improve. He decided to mention it at this visit because the doctor asked him if he had any other concerns.

The endocrinologist looked at him squarely in the eyes and said, "Dearest and wonderful gentleman, the symptoms that you are describing are not consistent with thyroid eye disease. Even if you do have mild thyroid eye disease, that is not the explanation for your symptoms, and it will not get better with the treatment of your hyperthyroidism," as was demonstrated by him being euthyroid on low-dose medications for years.

## A Crucial Discovery

Yes, as an endocrinologist, this doctor was clearly also an internist, but the practice was primarily endocrinology. The endocrinologist had to quickly look up the diagnostic workup for myasthenia gravis as a quick reminder so that they could order the appropriate initial test.

The doctor ordered an acetylcholine receptor antibody and sent him directly to the lab. The patient called a few days later for the results, and …yes…he had positive acetylcholine receptor antibodies and likely had antibody-positive ocular myasthenia gravis.

The doctor immediately called the neurologist, and he was seen that week and started on appropriate therapy and, to this day, remains asymptomatic and has never manually held his eyelids open again!

It is not uncommon that autoimmune disorders can co-occur in the same patient, so there are many stories quite similar to this one. You must have a high degree of clinical suspicion and a listening ear.

The cute part of this story is that if he had not mentioned it and if the doctor had continued to have perpetually morning appointments with him, the doctor would not have picked it up on clinical examination because the morning appointments would never have allowed direct observation of the drooping of his eyelids.

So again, listen to the patient and allow some time for open-ended questions in your encounters.

Somewhere along the way, I remember seniors saying, 'Trust no one'!! This was probably their way of saying, take your own history and examine your own patient!! This should always be done, at least to some degree, even if the patient you are meeting already has an established history.

## *The Power of Open-Ended Questions*

I can recall one more story that was shared with me that further illustrates the power of the open-ended question. A patient was being seen for her diabetes. At the end of the encounter, she was asked if there were any more concerns, or if overall, she was ok.

She proceeded to state that she was ok but that she needed another refill for her water pill because she ran out of it a few weeks ago, and she was having worsening swelling in her legs, and that now she had difficulty getting her shoes on.

The doctor asked her how long she had been on the 'water pill' and who had prescribed it. She did not recall when she started it, or who initially prescribed it. She would just get refills whenever she saw doctors.

She emphasized that she really needed it because her legs were swelling up so much. So, the doctor asked if she had any heart problems, chest pain, or discomfort, and she said 'no' to all of the above.

The doctor explained that it is not normal to have swelling whenever you stop a water pill and that she should be investigated for why she was having worsening swelling of her legs.

She asked if she could just get the prescription and follow up at a later date because she had been on the water pill for a long time and felt that she would be fine once she got back on the pills.

The doctor gave her a limited prescription with no refills and insisted that she see the cardiologist immediately to lead the investigation for the cause of her recurrent leg swelling. Fast forward to the follow-up visit with the doctor where the patient describes that she was seen by a cardiologist a few days after that visit.

She was evaluated with an EKG (ECG), echocardiogram, and other studies and was immediately referred for cardiac catheterization for the management of her silent coronary artery disease.

Had that doctor not really listened to the patient and acted in her best interest but had simply given her the refill like she asked for, he would have missed the opportunity to act and perhaps cause this patient to have a life-changing intervention which likely prevented a cardiac catastrophe.

He could have written the water pill prescription (which would have been so much faster) and told the patient to follow up in 4 months.

Instead, he listened when she told him that her legs were swelling and getting worse, and he took the extra three minutes to clarify what was going on and to make the appropriate referral, even though this was not the patient's intent when she was simply asking for her refill.

Of course, the patient was blown away and eternally thankful because she had absolutely no idea that she was in such trouble, and neither did the doctor.

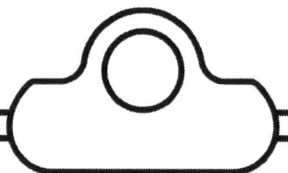

## BOTTOM LINE

Listen to your patients.

Listen to your colleagues.

Listen to the little voice in your tummy...your intuition.

Listen, listen, listen!!!

# ℞ ACTION PLAN

- [ ] Ask your patient an open-ended question even if you have addressed the reason for the consult. Yes, you're taking a chance, they could have a complaint that takes time to explore, but that time could save their life. If the complaint is something that's not in your area, it takes only a few seconds to refer a patient to someone else. If it is something that can wait, then table it for the following meeting and make the meeting a little sooner if needed.

# Chapter 6

# The Power of Eye Contact

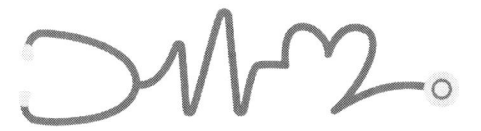

As we continue our deep dive into the importance of acknowledgment in physician-patient relationships, it is impossible to ignore the power of eye contact.

Generally, when communicating with a patient, or anyone for that matter, eye contact tends to make a significant statement. In fact, eye contact can communicate many things.

In my experience, establishing eye contact with a person tends to communicate the message that you are honest and comfortable with the information that you are relating.

Eye contact is a way of acknowledging that you are addressing them particularly, and it's a sign of respect. Eye contact allows you to read a person's body language and to receive nonverbal cues about how the interaction is going, from their perspective.

Eye contact assures the receiver of the communication that you are engaged with the interaction and that you care to confirm that they are indeed listening to you.

Finally, eye contact can be a very powerful means of communicating emotion and tone. There is definitely an art or skill to establishing the right amount and the right type of eye contact when communicating.

When eye contact goes wrong, this can have ramifications for the status of the relationship between the communicators. Too little eye contact can seem dismissive and too much eye contact, or staring, can be interpreted as aggressive or even make someone feel very uncomfortable.

These are the things that come to my mind when I think about the importance of eye contact and its role in interpersonal communication.

## *Balancing Eye Contact and Documentation*

While I was actively writing this book, I was super aware of when a patient made a comment to me about anything to do with our interaction or to do with their experiences with other physicians during clinical encounters.

I also found myself going through other standout scenarios in my mind. During my writing, I recalled an encounter that I had years earlier with a patient.

This patient was very uncomfortable initially, and to be honest, in the specialty of 'Obesity Medicine' where a significant portion of my patients struggle with excess body weight and the complications thereof, many of them tend to be very self-aware and very conscious and quite frankly, are in fear of judgment.

They do not know what to expect from the interaction and so their body language upon our initial engagement tends to be very closed. I am sensitive to this and am very careful to use very sensitive and nonjudgmental language and statements.

So, we spoke about her concerns and about the expectations for her management. Ironically, her primary concern was not actually her body habitus, but this came up as something that she wanted to address once we had resolved the primary issue for which she sought consultation.

I made the appropriate referral and gave her order forms for her imaging and blood tests that would be needed for her preop evaluation and for metabolic evaluation. We then planned to follow up later to discuss the results of the labs and ultrasound to finalize the surgical plan.

So, as we were leaving the room, she said to me that she found it difficult to believe that she could be so open with a doctor and ask all her questions and feel so comfortable.

She went on to say that she had sat through an encounter with a doctor recently who never once looked at her. (Obviously 'never once looked at her' was an impossibility, but I'm sure we get the picture).

Now the patient did admit that the doctor was covering for her usual physician and that the doctor spent most of the encounter flipping through the pages of the medical chart trying to piece together her medical history and make a plan for this visit.

However, the patient made the statement that she felt that the doctor really made no effort to connect with her personally or to see if there were any concerns to be addressed that day. She was lost flipping through notes and therefore immediately lost the confidence of the patient who mentally checked out at that point.

I feel that this doctor, if she didn't have any time to review the notes quickly prior to entering the room, would have been better off letting the patient know that he or she was covering for Dr. Indigo and then proceeding to take a brief history of patient's medical condition and medications and asking if there were any particular concerns today.

This could have been very concise, and also would have allowed Dr. White to meet the patient, have a quick conversation, and establish rapport.

Flipping through unfamiliar notes in front of a patient is seldom an effective approach and is quite painful, to say the least. A brief conversation allows you to observe the patient as you collect information, an opportunity that would be lost if you spent too much time flipping through notes.

Perhaps a brief review of the last encounter would have done the trick.

## *Practical Tips for Eye Contact During Patient Care*

Studies have supported the fact that nonverbal communication is of paramount importance in interactions with patients and in interpersonal interactions overall.

There are many aspects of nonverbal communication to consider, and while an appropriate gesture or touch can help to communicate empathy, and while the length of a patient visit also improves positive perceptions of the visit, eye contact seems to be one of the more powerful factors in conveying empathy to patients.

Eye contact in brief and regular intervals is recommended as a very effective adjunct to your verbal communication.

Overall, being mindful to try to provide at least a minimal amount of eye contact during a patient interview tends to establish that you are at least 'present' in the room for the moments that you are with the patient.

Remember that forced or unusually long episodes of eye contact can make any person uncomfortable in any scenario and can compromise effective communication or convey an unintended message. I am sure that many of us have been the recipient of awkward stares.

At times, if I am typing or reading through results or quickly reviewing something relevant to the conversation, I would ask the patient to excuse me for looking through the chart while we are speaking.

I would let them know that I am listening but wanted to review or type something while it was still at the forefront. Most times, the response is 'No need to apologize Doc!'

Acknowledging to the patient that you probably should be looking at them, reminds them that they are the reason for the interaction and that you are not just interested in numbers and reports.

Just keep the lines of communication as open as possible and be aware of the behavior of those present in the room, including you.[1,2,3]

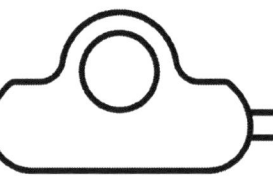

## BOTTOM LINE

Eye contact can send a message of empathy for your patient.

Appropriate eye contact can make you more likable.

Eye contact can allow you to gauge the patient's response to you and your message.

Try not to force your eye contact but try to develop it naturally.

# ℞ ACTION PLAN

- [ ] Work on establishing the right amount of eye contact when interacting with patients.

- [ ] Think about yourself and decide if this is something that you need to work on.

- [ ] Try to observe nonverbal responses from your patients and feel free to explore them if they indicate to you that a concern persists or that an explanation that you gave didn't clarify the matter for the patient.

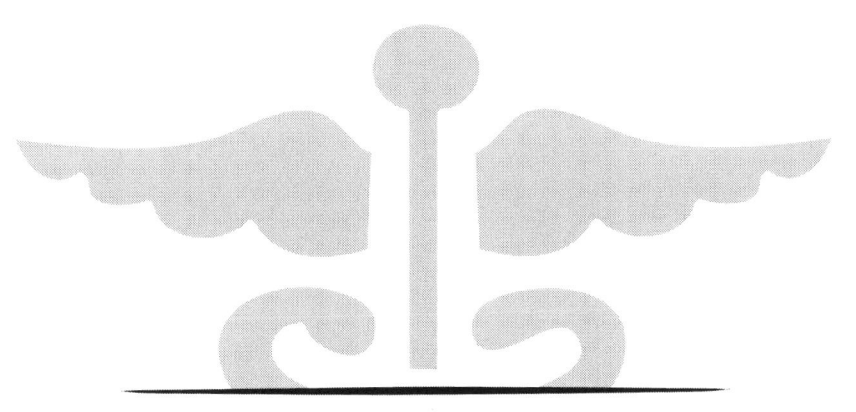

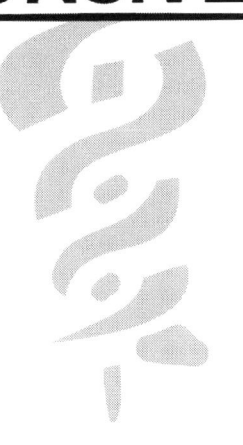

# SECTION 3
# RESPONSIVENESS

# REPONSIVENESS

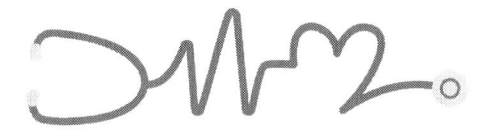

## "As you RACE through your Day, Don't Forget to C.A.R.E."

## "R" is for RESPONSIVENESS

The 'R' in C.A.R.E. refers to responsiveness. Many aspects of responsiveness are impactful in how your relationships will evolve. All interactions are affected by responsiveness, either negatively or positively, and so as we interact with those around us, let us consider the many dimensions of our responses.

Are you sensitive to the cues you receive from people, and are you aware enough to respond appropriately?

Are you able to pivot or redirect if the signals you receive tell you that your message is being lost, misinterpreted, or ill-received?

Do you care enough to even be aware of the signals that are being sent to you?

On another note, are you listening to the signals that your body is sending to you? The degree to which you respond to information dictates the degree to which you are transformed. Be open to transformation.

Let's explore, in the following chapters, several of the dimensions of responsiveness that impact our day-to-day interactions with patients and with ourselves, and let's see if we can be the master of our responses.

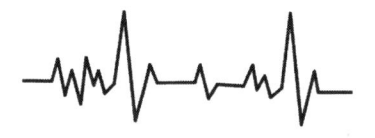

## Chapter 7

# The Power of Touch

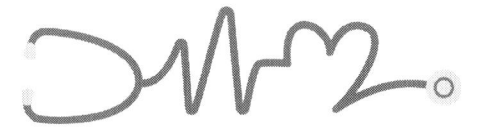

### *The Unseen Impact of Touch*

The power of touch could not have been exemplified more clearly than in the throes of the COVID-19 pandemic. During this time, we were isolated from family, friends, loved ones, colleagues, and patients. This has taken a toll on the way we interact with each other even today.

The power of touch in the doctor-patient relationship is a sacred one that is completely underutilized, in my opinion. Yes, there is a need to examine your patient as a part of your clinical evaluation, this touch is necessary and important, but this is not the touch to which I am referring.

The palpation of 'an abdomen' to detect an enlarged liver or the palpation of 'a chest' to identify the point of maximal impulse to screen for cardiomegaly are useful clinical tools that really can make a patient feel quite objectified, especially when the medical student displays unbridled excitement to have palpated his first 'liver'!

Think about being the mother of a child with large polycystic kidneys who is in the children's ward, whom all the medical students come by to examine. They are (visibly) excited to ballot a kidney; but imagine a mother feeling like people are more interested in examining her child than helping him.

These medical students are not bad people, they are honing valuable and essential clinical skills, but at the same time must be taught to develop and refine their human skills, because the kidneys that they are examining belong to a patient, a person, someone's child, and they should ask permission to examine the child and learn to be sensitive to what is going on in the life of the parent and the child.

## *Beyond Clinical Touch: The Human Connection*

So yes, examining a patient and clinical touches are a part of the patient interaction, but what I am referring to is the 'human' touch.

The pat on the shoulder, the handshake, or the touch on the upper back when someone is bent over in tears after receiving some bad news or is done relaying a difficult story to you.

If this person in this room has opened themselves to you, their physician, in such a way that tears are the result, then the appropriately placed touch can bridge the emotional and physical gap between you and the patient and make them feel that they are not alone in the current moment.

Even in biblical times, Jesus delivered his healing through touch in many instances.

## *Healing Beyond Medicine: The Role of Human Touch*

A simple touch (after the application of hand sanitizer nonetheless) can convey a message that simply says to the patient... 'I am here with you'. Imagine the specialist attending patients in an STD clinic.

I remember rotating through the infectious disease clinic. It is such a vulnerable setting in which to be seen as a patient. Often, the patients can feel isolated and judged. A lot of times they are hard on themselves, and their body language conveys that they are preparing to be judged and scorned.

This is seldom actually the case, but a posture of contrition is often what greets you. Walking into the room, washing your hands, and shaking the hand of or touching the shoulder of an 'HIV-positive' patient as you introduce yourself can change his life.

Stigma, misconceptions, shame, guilt, and negative personal experiences may cause a person living with HIV to be extremely protective of this information for fear of being mistreated, even by healthcare professionals.

In this particular scenario, this pat on the shoulder is a loud and clear signal that 'you are accepted, and you are a person, and I care about you, and I want to take care of you, and yes...I am willing to touch you!'

Think about how powerful this is, especially on the backdrop of this patient's possible past experiences. Go beyond the knowledge...and impart healing with your human touch. You have more power than you could ever imagine!!!

Take it from me...this patient notices, appreciates, and craves your human touch. Unleash your power to heal beyond prescriptions.

## *Embracing Empathy: The Power of A Touch*

There are volumes spoken with an appropriately placed 'human' touch. When I usher a patient into the room, I may give a quick pat on the shoulder and say 'welcome in' or I may shake a person's hand if that seems to be a preference for that patient.

Honestly, I usually let my gut guide me as to how to physically interact with a patient, if at all, outside of the physical examination. But this requires your willingness to show to your patient that you were a human being before you were a doctor.

Sometimes in the training for, and in the practice of medicine, we learn to distance ourselves from our patient's situations. This can be protective in some instances, given the number of sometimes unfortunate, challenging, and sad situations you can encounter on a daily basis, as a physician.

But with a certain degree of control, you can allow yourself to connect with your patient.

As I was contemplating this topic and writing my thoughts and experiences, thinking about how my comfort level regarding my physical interactions with my patients has influenced some of my physician-patient relationships, it occurred to me to search the literature to see if there were any published objective writings on the topic.

Not surprisingly, the question of the role of touch in medicine was not unique to me. There have been several writings on the topic.[1,2,3,4]

While a systematic review of the literature on the subject of the role of touch in the practice of medicine, and the perceptions of patients and physicians regarding its role, is beyond the scope of this current project, I must say that the topic of physical touch in the clinical setting has been examined by several studies and from several angles.

What is interesting is that regardless of culture, socioeconomic background, and race, the results of these studies tend to confirm that appropriate physical interaction is welcomed by most patients.

When considering the sex of the physician, the sex of the patient, the religion of the participants in the studies, and many other factors, once one has taken into consideration the general cultural roles and preferences, there is still a tendency for an appropriately placed and timed touch to be perceived as a gesture of hope, camaraderie, or respect.

Some patients even perceived an appropriate non-examination touch from the physician as healing, comforting, cordial, sympathetic, and empathetic. These touches were generally welcomed.

In general, commonly accepted sites of such a nonclinical, though therapeutic touch, would be on the upper arm, shoulder, and upper back. There was some variation in who would perceive a touch on the hand as welcomed or not, but if you live and interact with a community of patients, then societal norms will probably not be lost on you.

## *Professional Touch: Finding the Balance*

What am I saying? I am saying that when you become comfortable with yourself, with your degree of professionalism, your degree of medical knowledge, your patient, your clinical scenario, and your practice setting, don't be afraid to let interpersonal communication include the nonverbal interactions that can sometimes be more powerful than verbal ones.

This requires you to use not only your clinical judgment but also your cultural sensitivity, your mutual respect, your religious awareness, and sometimes your plain old 'Spidey Sense.'

## *Navigating Boundaries: The Ethical Consideration of Touch*

Now, obviously, we are not talking about unwelcome physical interactions or inappropriate ones, or about physical interactions that can be reasonably perceived in any manner other than as respectful and empathetic. If you are in doubt, then refrain from such an interaction or invite a chaperone into the interaction.

Of course, the touch that is deemed appropriate will be affected by the specialty in which you are practicing medicine.

This will be different for a gynecologist versus a pediatrician as these patient populations are clearly ones that can be considered vulnerable in any scenario, especially if there is a gender difference between the patient and the physician.

So, when it is appropriate and necessary, use a chaperone, then you can exercise the appropriate discretion when it comes to the physical interactions with your patients, including clinical physical examinations.

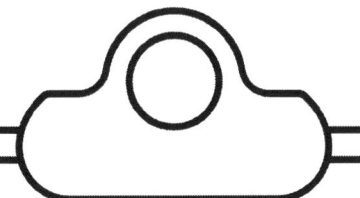

## BOTTOM LINE

With the appropriate reading of interpersonal cues, it is ok to touch your patient outside of the clinical exam.

An appropriately placed touch may make you stand out when compared to another doctor who may appear socially awkward or detached when faced with a patient in distress.

A carefully placed and appropriately timed touch can create a very special physician-patient bond and can communicate empathy.

# ℞ ACTION PLAN

- [ ] Think of a clinical scenario when you could have imagined using a personal touch appropriately to communicate empathy to a patient more effectively than you did.

- [ ] Think of a time when you did not use a physical touch to interact with a patient when it was appropriate not to do so. Continue to act appropriately when it comes to these scenarios and don't force a non-clinical touch in an awkward manner to try to improve your skills in this area. The appropriate moment will present itself again, and when it does, always proceed within your degree of comfort.

# ℞ ACTION PLAN

- [ ] Remember that the practice of medicine is exactly that, A PRACTICE. Each occasion to interact with a patient provides an opportunity to learn and improve yourself and to prepare for a better future interaction with that patient or with another patient.

## Chapter 8

# The Power of Effective Communication

The ability to effectively express an idea, and to have the receiver of that idea obtain the intended message, and then confirm such receipt, is the holy grail of communication, in my view.

When it comes to communication, we know from our introduction to communications courses in college, if we took one, that the effective conveyance of information from one person to another is wrought with potential 'noise'.

### *Encountering Communication "Noise"*

Noise is anything that occurs from the moment you speak your sentence to the moment that the patient hears the information and begins to understand what you are saying.

Noise can even occur during the closure of the communication loop, where the receiver would give a response to the received information, whether verbal or otherwise.

Noise can be the literal buzzing of your cellphone, or it could be figurative. Noise can represent anything that could serve as an impediment to the receiver of your communication actually tuning in to hear, understand, or properly interpret your message.

You must take into consideration the noise that exists in your communication environment and be willing to continuously survey the landscape if you are to communicate effectively on a consistent basis.

## *A Lesson from a Patient Encounter*

I remember a particularly hilarious encounter with a patient. I believe that she may have been coming to me for evaluation and management of hyperthyroidism.

Let's use hyperthyroidism for the purposes of this story. She had been referred by her primary doctor, and I took a great and thorough history. Any medical student would be proud of the painstaking detail that went into my history taking that day.

So, anyway, we went on to have a physical exam which was also relatively thorough, but definitely focused on the findings consistent with hyperthyroidism. My typical style is to explain plainly the diagnosis and what is happening with them physiologically to explain their clinical symptoms.

Then I would discuss the different treatment options with a patient and briefly outline the potential risks and benefits of each option. Then I would go on to ask the patient what they would like to do or how they would like to proceed.

I do have a cadre of patients who prefer a more paternalistic approach, and they would respond in a manner similar to the following: 'You are the doctor, you went to school to do this, so I will do what you recommend!'.

My older patients definitely tend to tell me to just give them what they need, tell them how to take it and tell them when to follow up.

More tech-savvy patients come to the consultation with printouts, AI recommendations, laptops, articles, notebooks, and textbooks. They send podcasts and email articles and all manner of things.

Now, to be fair, I have learned a thing or two from a patient or two.

Surprisingly, however, they generally don't have many questions after my brief anatomy, physiology, pathology, and pharmacology mini-lecture which precedes the 'How would you like to proceed?' question. I find it easier to answer some questions before they arise.

After many years in clinical practice, you tend to be able to anticipate most of the common questions that patients have with regard to certain diagnoses, and you can leave room for the other questions that an individual may have after.

Well, this fine day, after my usual lecture, I turned to the young lady, and I asked her 'What would you like to do?' Her eyes opened as if she was currently witnessing horns growing from my head in real time.

Out of those horns flew a polka-dotted flamingo on the left and a two-headed ostrich on the right. She folded her arms, and her body language completely shut down. She was aghast.

She paused for just a moment then said to me (In the best Bahamian dialect that I can muster up at the time of this writing) ... 'Vel what kind 'ah' foolishness dis is? I done pay all dis money to see the so-called specialist, and she ga look at me in my eyeball an ask MEEE what to do?? Well, I ga have ta tink bout dis one!!" (Translation... I spent all of this money to come to see the 'so-called' specialist ...and she doesn't have a clue how to handle this, so she asks me, the patient, what to do. I will have to think about this. (This doctor clearly does not know what she is doing if she has to ask me what to do.)

As she packed up her stuff and proceeded toward the door, I thought it futile but felt obligated to try to explain that I was simply giving her options given that I had laid out several of them for her.

Needless to say, I never saw that patient again. She returned to her primary care physician. I took that as a very powerful learning opportunity for myself. It was hilarious in retrospect, but actually quite unfortunate. I believe I have shared this story with only one person before now.

## *Adapting Communication Styles*

What is the bottom line here? Know your audience and read the room. Pay attention to your patient. Adjust your communication to fit the receiver.

She gave me many cues throughout my discourse that she was not particularly interested in my explanations or that she simply didn't really follow the medical things that I was trying to walk her through.

At any point, I could have (and should have) stopped and said to her, 'You have hyperthyroidism, you need to take these medications, get this ultrasound, and see me in 7 weeks. One week before you come to the office, go and get these blood tests so that we can see how your thyroid levels are improving. You should start to feel better in about a week'.

The encounter would have been much shorter and much more effective and would have met her needs. Instead, I lost a patient because I didn't adjust my style to meet her where she was.

Every patient encounter is an opportunity for your patient to learn something from you and for you to learn something from your patient. Sometimes what you learn is about yourself.

If I had allowed her to close the loop of communication, by acknowledging her signals that what I was doing was lost on her, or not what she desired from the encounter, I would have pivoted and rescued that encounter from disaster.

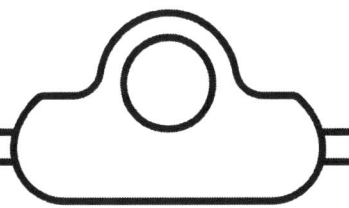

## BOTTOM LINE

Pay attention to your patients. Many times, their responses will clue you in regarding your effectiveness.

Change your approach if you are not having a successful interaction and are not meeting the needs of the patient.

Your 'style' does not work on every patient and for every encounter. Be aware of this and be present in the room and ready to take action to change the direction of the interaction if needed.

# ℞ ACTION PLAN

- [ ] Think about a time when you did not communicate effectively with a patient.

Think about the factors that lead to this lack of effective communication.

Were you very tired?

Did you just want to hurry and finish the clinic that day?

Were you distracted by the presence of another person in the room.?

Think of ways that you can improve on being wholly present in the encounter, even when the conditions are not ideal.

# ℞ ACTION PLAN

☐ Think of a transition statement you could make if you see that you are losing the patient in your attempt to communicate. Perhaps you can say, 'would you like me to try to explain that differently.'

You could say... 'before I continue is there anything specific that you would like to ask?' ..the patient might say to you... 'is there a medication that I can take to get better?'...and this is telling you that they want their prescription and their follow up appointment.

It's probably time to wind down.

Remember to pay attention to the part of the communication loop that is coming TOWARD you!!!

# The Power of Effective Communication

## *Part 2: Adapting Communication to Patient Needs*

On the other end of the spectrum is the patient who is eternally grateful for your willingness to communicate with them. When you take a little time to help patients understand what is going on and do things as simple as explaining what the pill you are prescribing for them is intended to treat, the physician-patient relationship is further cemented.

These are the patients who will bring their sister, mother, cousin, aunt, and best friend to see you. The act of effective communication can cause a patient to feel as though you are the first doctor to actually listen to them. The reality is, you just might be. The patients with whom you communicate well will try to come to you for everything because they trust you, they like you, and they feel like they know you!

These are the patients that when you refer them to another specialist, go for the consultation and then follow up with you shortly thereafter either bearing the original prescription of the recommended medications from said specialist, or the unopened box of the prescribed medications that they picked up three weeks ago, but refused to start until they had a chance to bring them to you.

Then they come with all the questions that they should have asked the specialist that you referred them to. You have to explain to them that the reason for the referral in the first place was that you don't know the answers.

When you continue to master the art of communicating well with your patients, they will decide that 'YOU' are their doctor, and that they will not do or take anything until you have seen it. This is a great responsibility, and you do have to politely redirect them to those more qualified than yourself to discuss matters when appropriate to do so.

This scenario may be different for someone who actually is the primary provider, but of course, I speak from the perspective of a subspecialist who chooses to practice her sub-specialty almost exclusively.

Effective communication does not have to be long-winded. We are all pressed for time, and I don't want you to believe that I am advising that you spend extended and impractical amounts of time with each patient. You can't!! Depending on your practice setting, you may not even be in control of the amount of time allotted for each patient encounter. What I am telling you is to make the most of each encounter.

## *Streamlining Patient Encounters*

Some of us are very limited in our encounter times, and if employed, we may have very little latitude when it comes to our schedules. So, in a 15-minute follow-up visit, we have to be very problem-directed and focused, so we have to learn to become very efficient and streamlined in our interactions.

Given the burden of documentation during the visits, the widespread use of electronic medical records, and the continued use of written notes, some of us are trying to document while we see patients, and this can lead us to spend more time looking at the screen and checking 'best practices' boxes than actually looking at our patients.

You should try to come up with a formula that works for you and your specialty and your practice setting that allows you to streamline your process. It will vary sometimes when you have a surprise, but for the most part, it can enhance your efficiency. I am honestly still working on this. Perhaps you can greet your patient and ask if there is any particular concern today.

Resist the temptation to interrupt within the first 15 seconds and allow the patient to speak uninterrupted for just a few minutes while you pay attention and give the appropriate amount of eye contact. Actively listen and then give your affirming touch. All of this can be done in 5 minutes. This leaves you a little time to delve into any complaint that might have been brought up.

You can do your focused clinical exam and then review medications and changes quickly, and briefly review the plan of action with the patient, and get up and walk them to the door where they can wait outside for their prescription and written directions. You can also quickly document in these three minutes, while the patient awaits their documents. In this quick follow-up, you made eye contact, listened to your patient, engaged in a non-clinical physical interaction, and came up with a plan all while not looking at your watch.

Even though we are rushing, we try not to let the patient feel like we are rushing, by avoiding obvious cues that we are rushed. Sitting down, even if only for a few minutes, communicates powerfully to the patient that you are present with them in the clinical encounter and that you have time (even if only very little) to listen to them.

If I am rushing, or late, I sometimes even state that...'OK, Mr. Black, all of my attention and energies are currently focused in this room. How can I help you today?'. The art of medicine has to be a little more intentional now, with the burden of documentation placed on practitioners and the new challenges posed by practicing medicine in a virtual space.

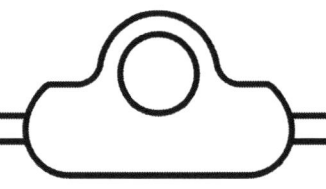

## BOTTOM LINE

Communicate well with patients.

Be intentional.

# ℞ ACTION PLAN

☐ Consider one thing you can implement to help you streamline your clinical process while implementing some of the tools to communicate to your patients that you are present with them in the clinical encounter.

☐ Think of one thing that you can implement to connect with your patient.

# ℞ ACTION PLAN

☐ Try to streamline your documentation process and be as concise as possible while still being thorough enough to capture the important information. This again is a challenge for me as I can be longwinded in my conversation and also in my documentation. Try to identify challenges that you have and develop a plan to mitigate the consequences of whatever inefficiencies that you can identify. Then implement and modify it as much as possible. I am working on being more direct in conversations and also on being more concise with documentation so that I can actually finish within a reasonable timeframe.

# The Power Effective Communication

## *Part 3: Communication in Sensitive Scenarios*

The power of communication is most relevant when one is awake and interacting with a person who is also awake.

Join me on a journey to the ICU, where I was consulted to assist with the management of a patient who had abnormal thyroid function tests. This was not the reason for her admission or for her subsequent respiratory failure, sedation, and intubation, which prevented me from meeting this young lady in an awake and non-sedated state.

I reviewed her chart and then entered the room to see the patient and to check the monitor. She was peacefully asleep, eyes closed, sedated, intubated, and mechanically ventilated. I introduced myself to her as Dr. Parker and proceeded to explain that I would be listening to her lungs and heart. While holding her hand, I quietly informed her that I would be feeling her pulse. Then I told her that I would just gently feel her wrist and touch her pulse.

Finally, before leaving, I mentioned that I would like to feel her neck to make sure that her thyroid gland was not obviously or palpably enlarged. Obviously, the exam conditions were not ideal, but they would suffice for the time being. I told her that I was an endocrinologist and that I was called because the team had done some blood tests that revealed that her thyroid function tests were abnormal.

I also told her that given that there was no reported history of thyroid disease in her, and given that her labs were consistent with thyroid hormone changes that occur in patients who are critically ill, I didn't believe that she had an organic thyroid problem and that I would not be initiating any medications for thyroid hormone abnormalities.

I told her that I would send off a special blood test and that I would trend her thyroid hormone levels intermittently because she had a central line and therefore would not have to get repeated sticks. I told her that I would be by tomorrow and the following days to check on her progress. She continued to be managed appropriately by her primary team for the underlying condition.

## *A Squeeze of the Hand*

Prior to going into the room on day two, I asked the nurses if there had been any changes and I was advised that she remained the same and was not responsive to verbal or tactile stimuli. There was no clinical deterioration. This was good. I figured I would just 'pop' into the room and say goodnight. So I did, and I held her hand and told her that her team was working very hard to help her through this difficult time and that we would be doing everything in our power to treat her well.

I told her that I was praying for her too. I told her that we and the nurses in the ICU would watch out for her. Then I told her I had to leave. As I held her hand, I asked her to squeeze my hand. I did indeed feel a very feeble squeeze of my hand but it was not reproducible. I carried on with my daily rounds and eventually, she started to improve with some flexion of hands and feet on command per the nursing staff.

She remained intubated and was intermittently sedated if she became excessively agitated throughout the course of the day.

As far as her thyroid hormones were concerned, they were abnormal because of her critical illness, and this is considered to possibly be a physiological response not requiring pharmacologic intervention. We would expect them to return to normal once the critical illness is resolved and we would follow them to confirm that they did.

So, after a few days of having been away, I returned to check on her and to see how she was doing. She had, by that time, been extubated and was being managed on the general medical floor awaiting transfer to a long-term inpatient rehab facility.

I decided to walk into the room. I knocked on the door and walked in and another person was sitting in a chair at the foot of the bed. I looked at the patient and her guest and asked, is this the room of Ms. Brown!!

## *Recognition Beyond Sight*

The patient looked at me and said, 'Good evening, Dr. Parker, how are you doing!! I recognize your voice and it's so nice to finally see you and meet you!!' Of course, I was frozen for a few seconds, but I had to maintain my composure. I can feel the 'goosebumps' running down my arms and back and the back of my neck as I write this story to you.

It must be remembered that I had never had an actual conversation with this patient, and she had never seen me (as far as I know). So, I was preparing to introduce myself to her and I was not prepared to be addressed by my name by someone whose previous encounters with me were solely with her having been intubated, sedated, and ventilated.

So maybe she did squeeze my hand. Maybe it wasn't my imagination, as I must admit, I began to entertain the possibility that I had imagined it. So, what am I saying, always speak to the person as if they can hear and see you. Perhaps they can, and even if they can't, speak to them the way that you would want someone to speak to your nana. Be gentle and compassionate.

## The Power of Attentive Care

We have all heard the story of the patient undergoing surgery who was anesthetized and chemically paralyzed but recalls hearing entire conversations about them from the operating room staff while they were 'under'.

I remember hearing of a patient who expressed such grave disappointment when she recalled a recent surgical experience. She described how she had been put to 'sleep' for a surgical procedure and recounted how she heard a team member in the operating room say, 'Just look at her, she is too big, who is supposed to lift her onto this table, I'm most certainly not doing it!'

She said that at that point she could not move or speak but wanted to say, 'Well, let me lift myself then'. She faded away shortly thereafter but will never forget how it felt to be spoken about in that manner and have no power to respond to it, to change it, or to walk away. It was a bitter experience, and she hopes that she will never have to seek 'care' at that institution again.

As a non-surgeon and non-anesthesiologist, I will not likely encounter this type of scenario (unless as a patient) and would not take the liberty of discussing the details of anesthesia awareness as I am not duly qualified or experienced to do so. But if these conversations are rude, demeaning, derogatory, and disrespectful, this could lead to a sense of betrayal, loss of trust, and even litigation.

Are a few jokes and inappropriate remarks worth that? This person trusts you ultimately, so try to resist the temptation to engage in 'O.R.' banter, which could compromise your integrity and otherwise undermine you personally and professionally, no matter how tempting it may be.

We are all humans so there is always the temptation to engage. But do your best to resist this. The particular scenarios that you will encounter will vary quite widely depending on your specialty, but the principles discussed in this writing are all applicable in some way.

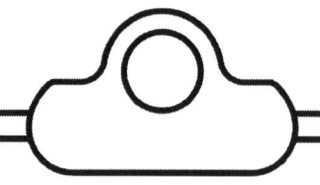

## BOTTOM LINE

Be respectful of patients, regardless of their state of consciousness.
If you find this hard to do, then be silent.

# Rx ACTION PLAN

☐ If you work in a critical care setting or you are asked to consult in one, greet the patient and introduce yourself to the patient when you enter the room and say goodbye when you leave. Touch the hand of the patient briefly before you leave, if appropriate. This may feel weird if your patient is comatose or sedated and you have never done it before. It will get easier. If you have not been in a coma or other altered state of consciousness, then you probably can't relate to how it feels, or speak authoritatively to the possible effects of someone speaking positive words to you or speaking words to you at all, while in such a state.

# CHAPTER 9

# The Power of Trust

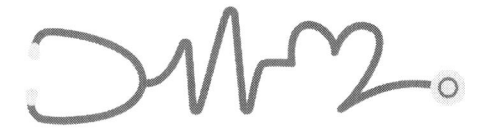

Trust, in the physician-patient relationship, is a delicate and necessary ingredient. When it comes to trust in this context, there are many dimensions.

The element of trust that I am going to address in this chapter relates to the element of implied confidentiality, which is one of the greatest facilitators of honesty on the part of a patient. When a patient feels that what they are about to tell you is private and confidential, it can change the dynamic of that relationship.

### *Confidentiality in Small Communities*

Now, this may seem obvious to one who may have trained in a system where a 'HIPAA' or confidentiality violation could cost you your job, reputation, license, and quite possibly your career, and it may seem insulting that I would think that it needed to be addressed.

But things are different when you live and practice in a small community.

There may be times when you see a sibling of someone that you know, or perhaps a spouse or significant other. Sometimes you may encounter multiple members of the same family, and none of the parties know that they have a doctor in common.

Even more interesting is that you may be tasked with the blessing and burden of being involved in the care of your own family member.

This latter scenario is generally discouraged for many reasons but can be virtually unavoidable when there are no other, or few other physicians with your particular specialty nearby.

## *The Unspoken Boundaries of Professional Integrity*

In this scenario, I have seldom had to state, that "for the record, the goings-on in this clinical encounter are between me and you alone." I may have said it once, not to someone related, but even the act of saying it for me was uncomfortable because, for me, it was automatic. I have never said that to another patient because I live it.

This sort of compartmentalization comes rather naturally to me, but for others, it might not. In small cities or on small islands, patients might refrain from seeking care locally because they may not, as we say, want all their business on the street.

Unfortunately, this is an actual concern, as it is possible that one might mention casually that another person is a patient of theirs. Now, this does not necessarily mean communicating what ails the patient, but that information alone communicates volumes, and I believe that that information in and of itself communicates too much.

Calling in a prescription while in a public place is a form of divulging patient information. You never know who is listening, step outside or move to the corner to complete such a call.

The dinner table is not the appropriate place to discuss the medical matters of someone who is a mutual acquaintance, or of anyone for that matter, certainly not if they are actually identified.

Discussing the medical situation of a patient with another doctor, who is not involved in their care directly, is inappropriate. My being a doctor does not automatically make me privy to another person's health information.

If you need to discuss a case with someone to help you process the information, then protect the identity of your patient. Being a doctor does not give them a right to know someone's health information, even if they have access to such information.

The thing about trust is, that once lost or broken, it is very difficult, if possible at all, to regain. Honestly, I tend to forget much of the details of why I saw someone as soon as they left the encounter. I need my notes. Names are even worse, so keeping it confidential is super easy.

I remember seeing a lady in the hallway of the hospital one day, and she ran after me quite enthusiastically. She was so excited to see me and was actually a little hurt that I didn't recognize her.

She said, "Dr. Parker, don't you remember me?" And I stared at her blankly, she said to me, "Don't you remember, you incised the abscess on my bottom yesterday and I feel so much better!".

She was not speaking softly at all. I laughed and told her that she should not discuss her medical information so loudly in the hallway as people could hear and see us.

She said to me that she was so happy that she felt better she could care less, and that she would see me next week in the clinic for follow-up and she carried on walking by. Real story! I say this to say, very often the doctor is in clinical mode when seeing or examining you.

It is very unlikely that he has noticed (or remembered) that your nails were not painted or that your legs were not shaved when he saw you at the last visit.

Ironically, I tend also to apologize to the doctor if my legs are hairy or if I forgot to lotion. I guess it's automatic to be hyper-aware if you are being inspected or examined, even if you are a doctor.

## *Maintaining Confidentiality Amidst Familiar Faces*

I am often tasked with patients who were referred to me by friends, other patients, siblings, or their parents and often they would say, "I sent my friend to see you," and they would call the name and ask if I saw their friend yet.

While most times I can't actually recall the name or if I actually saw them, I usually smile and say, "Now you know that I can't share any of that information with you." And typically they would say "I know doc" or they would say, "She told me she already saw you," and I would smile and leave it at that or say that it was great to meet her and that we got along very well.

But what this patient is now assured of is the fact that I am also not discussing their matters with other people either. Imagine if I had freely told them what I and their sister or friend discussed.

That would be sending a very loud message that what we discuss in these meetings is up for conversation with other people. That's powerful, and while they may smile, they are now wondering how freely I would discuss their clinical concerns with other people, both known or unknown to them.

If my patients decide to discuss our clinical encounters amongst themselves, that's completely up to them, but I am not at liberty to discuss our matters with other people, even if they are related.

Even when given permission, unless they attend the visit together, I would not discuss matters with patients who are acquainted with each other or who referred each other to me for management.

We must remain vigilant in protecting our professional integrity because it's easy to lose and oh so difficult to repair.

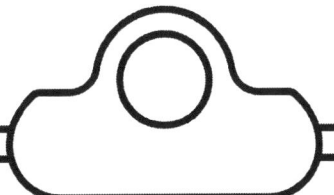

## BOTTOM LINE

Patient confidentiality is a matter of priority.

Remember not to discuss patient matters in public.

If called by the ER, the family, the pharmacy, etc., then step away from the crowd and remain aware of your surroundings as you discuss patient matters. You never know who's listening. It's a matter of trust.

If you think that a patient could be better served by another physician or specialist, refer the patient.

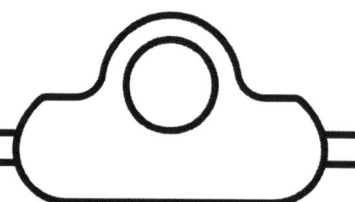

## BOTTOM LINE

If a patient sees you for consultation and you need a second opinion, or you need to run the scenario by your colleague, it's NOT ok to just identify the patient, because that patient came to you for help, not your colleague... and your colleague being a doctor does not automatically make it ok for you to give them someone's private health information.

This is difficult in a small society but it's just as true.

A lack of actionable consequences for breaches in confidentiality does not make it ok.

Ask the patient if it is ok to discuss the matter with a colleague.

# ℞ ACTION PLAN

- [ ] If you are in the habit of discussing patient information casually....STOP IT!!

- [ ] If you need an opinion or just need to vent, then de-identify the information.

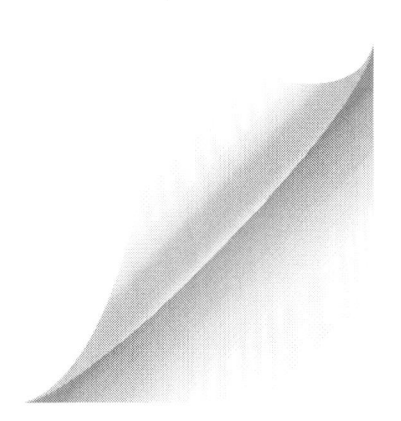

## Chapter 10

# The Power of Referring

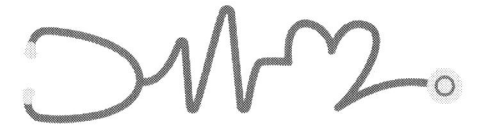

The power of referring is an extension of the power of trust. When a patient presents themselves to you for your opinion, or for your recommendations for their management, they trust that several things are true. They trust that who you represent yourself to be is actually who you are.

When you give a recommendation and guide a patient in a therapeutic choice, they are relinquishing their will, so to speak, and trusting yours. They are under the impression that you are making a well-informed decision and that you have their best interest at heart.

### *Refining Recommendations and Referrals*

Patients generally tend to be more comfortable when a physician is confident in their recommendations, but I find that patients are also happy when you have to look something up. It's all about how you frame it.

If you are not sure about how to proceed, then you can always excuse yourself and check the information. I would generally advise the patient that I'll take a minute to confirm what the guidelines recommend or advise them that I'm making sure that there were no material changes to the recent recommendations.

Patients like to hear the word 'guidelines'. It brings a sense of comfort that the message they are receiving is updated and cross-referenced, and that's because it is. There are conditions that are simply not common, and so refreshing your memory about how to proceed is precisely what you should do.

Don't feel pressured to make a recommendation that you are not certain about, or to give information on a topic that you haven't read since medical school 14 years ago. The pressure to appear knowledgeable can sometimes make you feel that any answer is better than no answer at all.

But the wrong answer is certainly not better than no answer at all. Take a few minutes and look it up. It's totally worth it. If you find that you are completely out of your comfort zone or specialty, then refer the patient to someone more qualified than yourself in that particular subject matter.

You should try to be familiar and comfortable with the knowledge and experience you have regarding a particular condition. This equips you to make solid recommendations.

## *The Significance of Specialization in Patient Care*

On many occasions, patients would try to pressure me into acting as a primary care physician for them, or they would present complaints and challenge me saying 'You're a doctor aren't you?!' This can definitely make for an awkward pause, but not for me.

My response typically goes something like this, I am excellent at what I am excellent at, and I am excellent at knowing what I'm not excellent at. I usually tell them that guidelines and recommendations in certain fields change rapidly and that those physicians practicing in particular areas generally keep abreast of changes in the specialties in which they are practicing.

I would say, I haven't looked at a knee in 14 years, do you really want me to give you 14-year-old non-specialized recommendations? At this point, the patient is usually quite happy to proceed to the orthopedic or rheumatologic specialist that I have referred them to.

Here again, communication with your patient and being comfortable with what you are comfortable treating can make this referral process run very smoothly. Don't take on challenges that you should not take on.

Don't be 'nice' or 'do it this one time'. It feels weird to be sending a patient with a complaint away, but do what is best for your patient and manage only what you are well qualified to manage.

I'm not just talking about your MD degree, which qualifies you, I'm talking about your exposure, experience, and comfort with the particular condition. It's ok to say NO!

It's not a sign of strength to try to treat everything, the converse is true, it's probably a weakness not to recognize when referring a patient is best for their well-being and for yours! Fear of 'losing a patient' by referring them, is not a reason to keep managing a patient sub-optimally.

Most subspecialists do not wish to assume primary care management of patients. They wish to optimize and treat specifically what the patient was referred for and to send the patient back to their primary physician for routine primary care.

In rural and geographically remote or isolated communities, you may well find yourself being the only physician for miles. Access to a specialist may actually be impractical or impossible. In these cases, pull up your bootstraps, look it up if you can, and carry on smartly doing the best of what is available for your patient.

In the absence of these circumstances, consider sending your patient for the opinion of a specialist. The patient will thank you!

Often, I get the question from a patient new to me, 'Why didn't they send me three years ago', and obviously answering this question can be quite difficult. I refer my patients to primary care specialists routinely and it is a luxury that I greatly enjoy.

## *Consultation Dilemmas: To Refer or Not to Refer*

The power of referring can also become relevant in discussions and relationships with colleagues.

I remember receiving a call from an internist late one evening. She called and gave the clinical scenario of a patient that she was co-managing. The patient had a neurosurgical condition and had developed a complication that was rather rare and unusual. The problem was that this complication was generally co-managed by multiple specialists because there was really no standard of care or guidelines.

In very specialized referral centers, the neuro-ICU would manage such a complication because by virtue of the volume of specialized patients that are referred to them, they would have the most experience. The condition was so esoteric that I was literally looking it up as she was speaking to me and, I had absolutely no experience in managing it and had never come across it in my training or clinical practice to date.

Honestly, other than looking up case studies and managing according to what I was reading, I didn't see how I could meaningfully contribute to the management of this patient and it made me very uncomfortable. I was uncomfortable coming on board because I really had no specific training in this area, and I was uncomfortable telling her that I was uncomfortable.

She was calling a specialist for a consultation and the specialist was about to tell her no. This was unheard of. I didn't want to come on board and struggle, but I didn't want to be seen as someone who couldn't handle such a case.

While I was reading (while she was on the phone) I saw where neurology and nephrology were usually contributing to the care of such patients, and this is what I suggested.

She was already waiting to hear the recommendations from the nephrologist so we agreed that she would see what he said and call back if needed. I literally lost sleep over this, and perhaps I should not have.

It might just be a personality flaw or characteristic. I'm sure I know other people who would simply have said that this is not my area and would have been quite happy to move on with their lives. I was not blessed with that gift, unfortunately.

So of course, rather than letting it go, the next morning I messaged her to find out how it was going, and she said that some things were improving, and some things weren't but that she was working with the nephrologist whose recommendations she had not yet received.

So, I advised her that I was reluctant because it was not an area of specialized knowledge for me, but that if her team was unable to make headway then they could consult me at that time.

Could this be a fear of not being consulted again? Could it be that perfectionism, which is often a personality trait of those who pursue medicine as a career, was stopping me from definitively saying no? Could it be that I did not want to look as if I didn't know something??

But honestly, she could look it up just as easily as I could and since I had nothing to add, should I really do the consult? In residency and fellowship programs, we generally don't have a choice.

If we are consulted, we see the patient and perhaps advise that it is not in our area, and we would leave our recommendations to consult the appropriate specialty and sign off. In private practice, I do have the luxury of declining a consult.

Perhaps this was the first time I encountered a consult that was worthy of declining and so navigating this was difficult for me. In retrospect, I do not regret it. I did feel a little funny the first time I saw my colleague after the 'event', but eventually this faded. They probably moved on immediately, but it took a while for me.

## *Guiding Principles for Navigating Complex Cases*

The above scenario is quite different from managing a rare condition that is within my specialty. Sometimes rare conditions will never be seen during training. You may or may not even read about them.

There may or may not even be guidelines to help you and you may have to rely on case studies, if you can find one. These, I am happy to deal with.

I have had to walk this lonely road before, and happily for my patient and myself; those case studies, my confidence, the patient's confidence in me, and our research led to a great outcome.

So, acting within your specialty, even if it is out of your comfort zone can be ok. But acting outside of your specialty and outside of your comfort zone can be risky, so tread carefully, and cautiously, and don't forget to 'look it up'!

Communicate effectively and be open and honest when you are dealing with colleagues and patients. Sometimes you will be in awkward and uncharted waters, there is no guideline for how to get through these tough scenarios, but my best advice, based on experience, is to communicate openly and honestly expressing your concerns and cautions.

Your colleagues and patients will appreciate it.

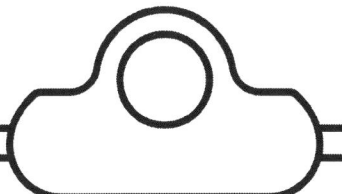

## BOTTOM LINE

Not every patient requires a specialist referral. Try to recognize those that do. It is not a sign of failure to be unable to help your patient meet treatment targets, but you do fail your patient when you continue along the same cycle while expecting different results.

If something is not in your area of specialization, you should probably let it be managed by someone else.

Know your limitations and learn to be comfortable that they indeed exist.

# ℞ ACTION PLAN

- [ ] When you see a patient with a complaint that is significantly outside of your comfort zone, if you have a specialist available to you, refer the patient.

- [ ] If you need help, refer to articles and guidelines, and colleagues to assist you. You are not expected to know everything, but you are expected to know what you don't know. Look it up if you must!

## Chapter 11

# The Power of Professionalism In Your Office

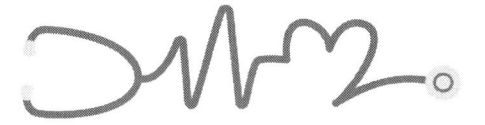

Long before a potential patient ever gets the pleasure of meeting you, they call your office. And long before they speak to you, they are speaking to someone on the telephone.

As a woman, a patient, a mother, a person, a human, a consumer, and someone who is very protective of my healthcare information, I can tell you that I have declined to make an appointment with physicians I have never met, based solely on the reception I received on the telephone.

The art of communication and customer service is paramount, not only for you but for all members of your staff.

From the custodian, who has no clinical responsibilities at all, to the reception staff, to the nurse or your physician assistant who may assist you with actual patient care and procedures; every single person that can be seen or heard by a patron, or potential patron, of your healthcare facility should have at least the most basic form of training in simple courtesy.

In many practices, appointment booking takes place online, and confirmations may be automated and computerized. In these cases, the first encounter may be the person manning the entrance to the facility or the receptionist at the front desk.

These people are your first line of defense. Make sure that they draw people in and do not push them away.

## *The Power of Professionalism Over the Phone*

I recall calling a gynecologist's office to set up an initial consultation. I remember hearing so much talking, giggling, and shouting in the background that I thought to myself, "Wow, this place sounds like a market."

In my mind's eye, I could see files everywhere, and I could imagine them handling my information very carelessly. While this was not necessarily the case, as I had never visited the practice or met the doctor or her staff, it was the impression I got, and I politely said that I had dialed the wrong number and hung up the phone.

The perceived environment is so important; a sense of professionalism must be maintained and portrayed at all times. It reassures a patient that they and their information will be handled with care and delicacy.

## *Ensuring Privacy and Professionalism in Practice*

Another encounter I remember was at an office where my lab order, given by the physician to the assistant to be stamped and returned to me, led to an uncomfortable situation.

The staff member looked at the lab order, must have recognized my name, then started to double-take at me and take a second look at the lab order to see what tests were being ordered.

She then looked me up and down and paused while staring at me as if to say, "Oh, now I see what is going on with you." The problem here is that her job was to stamp the form and return it to me.

The extra time spent looking at my information was not clinical in nature, and I could only imagine how she would comb through my results once they came in from the lab to see what was wrong.

Needless to say, I did not do those labs nor did I ever return to that physician's office. I sought care elsewhere. Staff members at all levels of the organization need to understand the critical importance of sticking to their duties and they should not go out of their way to interact with patient information.

Knowing that people who are not directly involved in your care can potentially access your information is already daunting enough, but seeing someone look you up and down and then look at your lab orders with curiosity while obviously making assumptions about you is inappropriate in a doctor's office.

## *The Significance of Staff Conduct in Patient Retention*

Remember that people have a choice when it comes to choosing a healthcare provider, and word of mouth, and these days, social media, can cause uncomfortable scenarios and experiences at your office to spread like wildfire.

This can sully the reputation of your practice and deter both existing and potential clients from seeking services at your institution.

This would be tragic, given that you are likely quite skilled at what you do, as evidenced by the fact that you seek to further develop yourself by reading and engaging with this work.

## *Leadership and Accountability in Healthcare*

So, remember, your staff is an extension of you, and they are very much a part of the experience that a patient has when seeking care from you.

Choose well and don't hold on to people who do not fit well with the flow and 'vibe' of your practice and space. The staff and team members that you choose to interview, select, hire and retain are either your choice, or they are your fault!!! When it comes to your team, good enough is simply not good enough. That's a lesson I learned from my recent readings, and it is such a powerful message.[1] If it's too much for you, then it's probably time to consider an HR professional.

It has prompted much introspection and will guide the decisions I make for years to come. It takes away the power of excuses and places the responsibility of your decisions directly onto you.

Another lesson I've learned from studying entrepreneurship is the concept of 'failing fast'. If something isn't working, pivot quickly and make a different decision.

Don't spend more time on a decision that isn't serving you or your vision. Acknowledge when it's not ideal and make another decision.

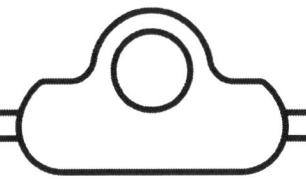

## BOTTOM LINE

Your staff plays almost as important a role as you do in the running of your practice, and in your ability to attract and retain patients.

# ℞ ACTION PLAN

- [ ] Take into consideration the behavioral tendencies of your staff and their personalities. Make sure that you train your staff to act in accordance with the behavioral standards that you wish to uphold within your organization. You may require help from a human resources professional. It's worth the investment because bad staffing can cost you.

- [ ] Listen to the feedback that you receive from clients. They are the reason that you are in business.

- [ ] No patients?... No practice!

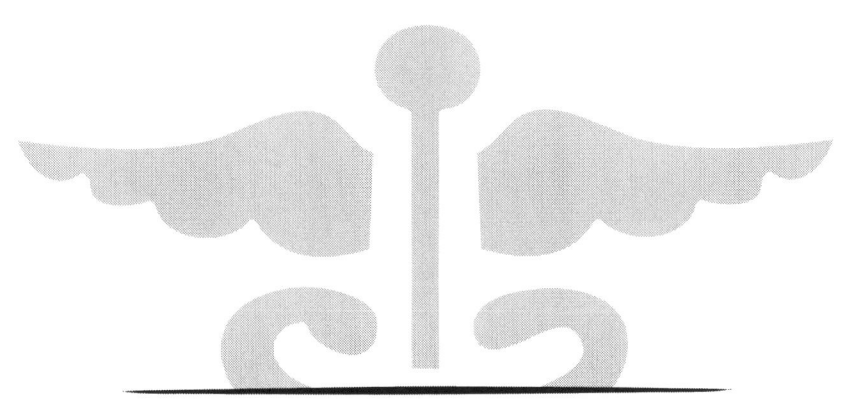

# SECTION 4
# ENGAGEMENT

# ENGAGEMENT

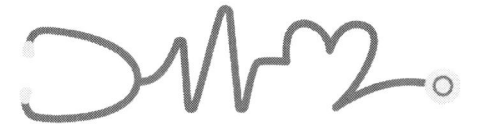

"As you RACE through your Day, Don't Forget to C.A.R.E."

## "E" is for ENGAGEMENT

In the final section of this book, we will explore themes of the process of engagement with your patients. When we engage with a patient, we try to form a connection that has bilateral meaningfulness.

The process of engagement speaks to meeting a patient where they are so that you can receive the message that they are sending to you.

Truly engaging a patient and attempting to actually relate to them and show empathy for their journey differentiates you from one who simply collects a list of signs and symptoms and generates a diagnosis and gives a patient a prescription and a plan, even if that prescription and plan are good.

Someone not engaged misses the fact that the patient cannot afford the prescription that they just wrote and entirely misses the opportunity to prescribe a generic alternative.

Being engaged speaks to being attentive and sensitive enough to navigate different scenarios and we will explore these themes in this final section of this book.

Finally, being engaged also speaks to the process of being engaged with your inner self, your spirituality, your hopes, your dreams, your aspirations, your disappointments, your triumphs, and how all these affect your day-to-day life and your interactions with those whom you serve.

Being engaged and honest with yourself allows you to address the concerns and challenges that may arise in your own life that can influence your interactions with others.

Now let's journey together one more time beyond the knowledge.

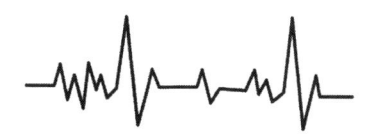

# Chapter 12

# The Power of Relatability

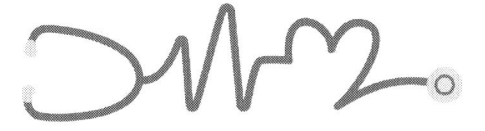

So, we are discussing in this book some of the many components of the physician-patient relationship and some of the things, which in my experience, and which also according to the literature, can help you to take your ability to relate to and care for patients, to an entirely new level.

The power of relatability can incite many connotations but the one that we will explore first is relatability when it comes to your ability to discuss a medical condition with a patient.

How good are you at expressing your concern to someone in a way that causes them to reframe their thinking and to accept something that they may have been in denial about for decades?

Let's discuss the good old 'silent killer', hypertension. It might be beyond the scope of this chapter to discuss the role that 'physician inertia', 'treatment inertia', or 'therapeutic inertia' plays in the management of hypertension, but we will touch on it very briefly now.

This inertia speaks to a tendency to 'watch and wait' or to 'see what happens' with regard to initiating antihypertensive therapy in patients who repeatedly have elevated blood pressure readings in the office.

I am not talking about malignant hypertension or symptomatic hypertension or blood pressure (BP) elevations that would be frightening to not address at the encounter, I am talking about elevated blood pressure that both you and the patient decide is elevated but 'not too elevated' or 'not that high'.

In this type of paradigm, the physician and the patient can leave hypertension untreated for years before finally deciding to initiate pharmacotherapy. Hopefully, there was some discussion about lifestyle recommendations and 'DASH DIET'[1], home BP monitoring, and other non-pharmacologic interventions.

What I am talking about in this chapter, is the resistance that the patient has to either accepting that he has hypertension (high blood pressure, HTN, elevated BP) or accepting that pharmacologic therapy is the right choice for him.

So, this scenario, for me, typically begins with me saying something like, 'Well, the blood pressure reading is elevated' and I would pull up the past few readings and say 'Looking at the trend, you have elevated BP that qualifies for a diagnosis of hypertension'. I think you should be treated for hypertension.

The thing is, I am seldom the primary physician and the visit to me that is the occasion for such a conversation is seldom for a primary complaint of hypertension. But it is difficult to repeatedly see a patient who has uncontrolled hypertension and not offer an opportunity for intervention.

## *Patient Perspectives on Treatment*

The patient, in response, almost always has a closing of their body language, an obvious resistance to or rejection of the idea of antihypertensives, or so called 'pressure pills'. The patient would advise me that their BP always gets a little elevated at doctor visits, or further, they would let me know what is going on that is causing the stress that is resulting in the elevated blood pressure that we are seeing today.

They do not have 'hypertension', their blood pressure is elevated because they are dealing with some stress at the moment. Now, we will not get into the definition of hypertension and the role of home BP monitoring or 24-hour ambulatory BP monitoring in its diagnosis.

Our patient, for the purpose of this discussion, has bona fide hypertension. He has advised me that he has heard that 'once you get on those things (referring to antihypertensive medication), you can't get off'. The next patient advised me that she does not want to be 'hooked' or 'dependent' on blood pressure medications.

Another patient said that he does not feel anything so he knows that his blood pressure is not that bad, another patient might say that she knows when her blood pressure is high because she can feel her head and neck hurting, so she knows that this is when she should really take the pills that her other doctor prescribed for her.

But she never really feels her BP so she generally does not need the medications. We have time for about two more reasons that patients resist taking blood pressure medications.

One popular deterrent is usually stated thus; ' doc, those pills have too many side effects man, I can't take that chance', and finally… 'doc, 'junior' might not work if I take those pills…and you know junior gat to be able to stand right doc?… right!?!'.

So, if you are a primary care physician, a general practitioner, a family medicine specialist an internist, an endocrinologist, a cardiologist, or a doctor in any other specialty really, you may well be familiar with these 'excuses' and you are either currently laughing out loud on nodding your head in agreement because you know exactly what I am talking about and you can see the face of your patient right now, or you are rolling your eyes or slapping your forehead with the palm of your hand saying to yourself 'I know right!?!'. Yes…I do know!

If you are a patient, then right now, there might be some silence and introspection, or you are in total agreement with the above sentiments. Doctors are not exempt from this mentality, and many forego treatment sometimes at the expense of their careers or lives. Doctors are patients too!!

After all, we are only people who went to medical school, we are not super-human. Not most of us, at least.

## *Addressing Medication Myths*

I am sure that in many ways, and on many occasions, you have discussed the risks of untreated hypertension with your patients, and you have assured them that there are many medications that will not interfere with (little man's) erections and that 'junior' or 'mini me' or 'maxi me' or 'anaconda' is more likely to be damaged by untreated hypertension than by the side effects of medications.

I sometimes find it useful to advise patients that medications indeed have POTENTIAL side effects and that in a study, if 8 people report something, then it must be reported as a 'potential' side effect and that it might not be very likely that they would experience that effect at all.

I advise them that every decision that we make, really, has potential risks and potential benefits, and that if the potential risks outweigh the potential benefits, then they should absolutely walk away from that option; but that if the potential benefits outweigh the potential risks, then perhaps they should consider it as a reasonable option and then give it a go cautiously.

Some, in fact, may respond to this, especially when I advise them that the risk of uncontrolled hypertension significantly outweighs the risk of a medication, which can easily be substituted for another one if a patient experiences an adverse effect.

This addresses the group of patients who think that their BP should be treated but are reluctant to try medication because of anxiety about the treatment itself. It's also sometimes very useful to point out that many common over-the-counter analgesics and other nonprescription medications have potential side effects, including bleeding, kidney damage, liver damage, and more, but that they take those medications without a second thought if a part of their body hurts.

Pain relief trumps not treating to prevent a 'hypothetical' complication in most instances. The first liver transplant patient that I ever encountered lost their liver function from overuse of an over-the-counter pain medication.

## *The Power of Analogies*

Let's discuss how we could possibly relate to a patient who does not see hypertension or high blood pressure as a problem that needs to be addressed in the first place.

This is a tough group because they are correct in most cases, in that they are completely asymptomatic and can continue with the activities of daily living with few impediments from hypertension, especially if mild or moderate. In most cases, hypertension is generally not painful, symptomatic, physically restricting, visible to other people, or bothersome in any way to the bearer of this elevated blood pressure.

So, the pressure to treat this abstract condition, which really is not bothering the patient in any consciously appreciable way, is not there, as far as they are concerned.

We all know that sometimes the first symptom of hypertension is a catastrophe (a stroke, heart attack, retinal bleed, visual impairment, or renal failure and the resulting need for renal replacement therapy), but these things are so 'far off' in a patient's mind and are not likely, in their view, to happen to them, because their blood pressure is 'not that bad'.

## *Visualizing Health Conditions*

So, the illustration that I often use is that I tell the patient to imagine that they are watering the grass with a hose. The water runs smoothly from the nozzle or opening and flows in a relatively calm manner depending on the water pressure.

Then I tell them to imagine that they want to water the hedge but that they really don't want to walk to the hedge or perhaps imagine that the hose is just a little short of the hedge, so they use their thumb to partially occlude the opening of the hose so that the water shoots out of the hose with so much pressure that if they accidentally directed that flow toward the flower patch, all the petals would fly off the flowers and the flowers would be destroyed by the pressure of the water coming out of the hose.

Then I advise them that their blood vessels are like tiny little pipes or hoses carrying blood from one area of the body to another, and that these vessels (or pipes) were not designed to carry fluid under such high pressure, and that over time the walls of the vessels can become weakened and even rupture under that constant elevated pressure which can lead to a bleed in the brain (a 'stroke').

Then I explain that the part of the brain that would normally receive blood and oxygen from the blood vessel that ruptured now has no oxygen delivery, and would die. The function of the part of the brain that died would be lost, for instance, if the part of the brain that controlled the movement of the left arm lost its blood supply when the vessel ruptured, then you would not be able to move the left arm. This is what happens with a (hemorrhagic) stroke.

Sometimes the blood vessel walls become thick over time, from withstanding so much elevated pressure. If the vessel walls become overly thickened, then they can actually narrow the vessel, block the flow through the vessel, and decrease blood delivery to parts of the brain.

This can starve parts of the brain of the blood supply that brings oxygen and cause an ischemic stroke. Elevated blood pressure can cause slow and also very sudden changes that are often irreversible and that many at times occur without warning.

Practically everyone knows what a hose is, and most people have used one and can relate to putting the thumb over the opening to cause an increased flow of water. Therefore, the relatability of this story when explaining hypertension tends to have persons quite willing to see that the risk of uncontrolled hypertension is unacceptable.

They have a visible picture, in most cases, of the force of that water leaving the hose and flying across the yard, and it's scary to imagine that degree of pressure tearing away at their blood vessels.

## *Connecting Conditions with Daily Life*

We can further extend this illustration to explain why we treat hyperlipidemia (high cholesterol) and diabetes.

When I speak to my patients about the complications of diabetes, I tell them that the blood vessels are like pipes and that in the same way that steel pipes were not designed to carry liquid rich in salt, blood vessels are not designed to carry a liquid that is rich in sugar. I would then ask the patient what would happen if a steel pipe were continuously exposed to salty water, and most people would respond that it would eventually get rusty.

So, in that vein, I would continue the explanation that the abnormal elevations of sugar in the circulation can cause damage, abnormal buildup and corrosion, clogging, and sometimes weakening and rupture of blood vessels.

Damage to, and sometimes rupture of these vulnerable blood vessels in the eyes, kidneys, and the nerves that supply the feet underlie the common complications of diabetes that lead to blindness, kidney failure, and nerve damage that can lead to diabetic foot pain, ulcers and infections, and amputations.

Patients are usually pretty silent by this time, and I continue to explain that when you have three processes (high blood pressure, high cholesterol, and high blood sugar) assaulting the integrity of the blood vessels in one body, then it is super imperative to be aggressive in protecting those blood vessels.

So, this is why, if you have diabetes and high blood pressure and also high cholesterol, which all compromise the integrity of the blood vessels, all while you feel nothing at all, then you are simply a 'ticking time bomb'.

Now, we don't have the power to control all of the events that occur in our lives, but if we have the power to make an intervention that could decrease our risk of cardiovascular disease or complications, then why would we not?

I can tell you, that bringing this home to patients with an illustration that they can visually relate to seldom fails to have a patient rethink their approach to protecting their blood vessels.

## *Simplifying Diabetes Management*

So, let's take the concept of relatability one step further for the diabetics. Before we even get to discussing the importance of protecting the blood vessels from sugar, patients sometimes ask, 'What is diabetes anyway?'

Diabetes is usually explained by me as follows; when you eat, chew, swallow, digest, and absorb your food, the nutrients eventually get absorbed from the gut and transported into the circulation. One of those nutrients is sugar. Sugar is found in obvious places like cookies, soda, juices, other sugar-sweetened beverages, candies, and sugar that you add to your tea.

Sugar is also found in foods that you may not realize (like in rice, potatoes, bread, crackers, pasta, corn, and grits) because these 'starches' and 'carbs' are broken down to sugar by the digestive process.

When these sugars enter circulation, insulin is the hormone responsible for escorting the sugar out of the blood vessels and into the cells of tissues where the sugars are used to supply energy.

Patients with prediabetes and type 2 diabetes are resistant to insulin and therefore their insulin does not work as well. Their pancreas compensates for this by producing more insulin and releasing it into circulation, but at some point, the pancreas is making its maximum amount of insulin and cannot further increase its insulin production in an effort to lower the circulating blood sugar levels.

At this point, sugar (glucose) levels in the blood start to rise, and these abnormalities can be detected on blood tests. This may be an oversimplification of the process, but it captures the main points in a relatable way.

So, the glycemic management of diabetes and prediabetes consists of three major tenets: first, try to decrease the amount of sugar that you are introducing into your body (dietary adjustments, fist-sized carb portions, avoiding sugar-sweetened beverages).

The next component is to increase the amount of sugar that you are burning (exercise). Finally, we can use medications to assist in improving the way your body handles glucose and insulin via varying mechanisms.

This seems cumbersome but does not actually take very long, and it brings patients up to speed relatively quickly.

Trust me, after doing it regularly, it rolls off your tongue, and patients have very few questions because you would have summed up most of the common questions that I get asked as an endocrinologist, even by patients who have been diabetic for years.

Now you are more than welcome to use my illustrations with your patients once you acknowledge its source as 'The KPC method'.

## *Empowering Patients Through Education*

One more thing that I find puzzling is the number of patients that I encounter with long-standing diabetes who have no idea what hemoglobin A1C is. This measure is one of the fundamental targets when it comes to decreasing the risk of complications in diabetic patients.

To simplify this concept, I try to break it down to the simplest terms so that anyone with any grade level of comprehension can understand it on some elementary level. The truth is that there need not be deep understanding.

A basic working knowledge of the targets that we have and why we have them puts your recommendations into some tangible context for the patient and makes the likelihood of adherence to recommendations more likely.

Typically, I would explain to a patient that hemoglobin is a component of your blood and that when this hemoglobin is exposed to sugar that is in your circulation, the hemoglobin turns into a sugary hemoglobin called hemoglobin A1C (HbA1C). We can calculate what percentage of your hemoglobin has been converted to this sugary HbA1C.

The higher the blood sugar level and the longer that those levels remain elevated, the more hemoglobin will be converted to sugary hemoglobin and the higher your percentage of HbA1C will be. The higher the percentage of sugary hemoglobin, the higher the risk of complications from diabetes, and that's why we try, in general, to keep this percentage below 7%.

What do you think the first question is that follows this explanation? That's right... 'Doc, what's my A1C level?' And just like that, this person has become fixated on this number and goes on to ask, 'What should I do to get my number down?'.

This interest alone is half the battle won. Patient 'buy-in' to why you are recommending what you are recommending is certainly an important factor in increasing the likelihood that he or she will adhere to the recommendations and even further, will start to do their own research as to what he himself, or she herself can change about their lifestyle to try to improve this number.

So now, your patient has a challenge, a target, and action steps and wants to know when is the soonest that they can recheck this number. In my experience, when you create something relatable for the patient, they have more confidence in their understanding of what is going on with them and they feel empowered to act, at least, for the moment.

Remember that long-term change requires reinforcement and encouragement and a nonjudgmental attitude when behavioral changes veer off course.

## *Navigating Long-term Patient Relationships*

During the course of long-term relationships with your patients, if you happen to care for individuals with chronic, non-communicable medical conditions, you can learn the art of meeting a patient where their needs lie and improving your patient engagement skills.

I typically have to remind my patients to think of our encounters as guard rails. Over time, patients can tire of regular visits, and understandably so. Also, they can sometimes get comfortable with their management regimens and start to delay appointments or skip them for months on end.

Sometimes they feel that they are doing ok that they can therefore forego the follow-up visit. Another common scenario is that they want to improve before they come back to the visit so that they don't 'get in trouble' lol. I try to reassure them that this is a 'judgment-free zone', and most of the time it is.

But the point of the meeting is to check in, review labs, and see where we are, and get back on track if we have veered off. If you do these three to four times per year, then you will be reminded to re-adopt the positive behavior changes that lead to initial improvements.

## *The Power of Storytelling in Medicine*

One more story before we move on to the next topic. This story quickly illustrates the power of storytelling in your efforts to communicate with your patients, and it also reiterates the need to find ways to break things down to patients in relatable and practical ways.

I remember a story of a patient who was grappling with a new diagnosis of lung cancer. He was a very young and functional 60-year-old man who went to the doctor for a persistent cough. He was eventually sent for an X-ray and further imaging and investigations.

Ultimately, he underwent an appropriate resection for his newly diagnosed lung cancer. He was referred to the oncologist who was counseling him about the risks and benefits of the recommended chemotherapy.

This patient, who was perfectly well just weeks before his diagnosis, couldn't accept that he had a disease that, all of a sudden, required chemotherapy that would turn him into a 'cancer patient'.

He refused to accept this and went on to explain that he thought that because the surgeon had removed the piece of the lung where the cancer was, he thought that he was cured and did not see why someone would try to give him chemotherapy.

The oncologist looked at him and asked him if he did any gardening, and the patient responded that yes, he did do gardening quite a bit actually. The doctor went on to ask him if he had ever weeded his garden.

The doctor then asked him what happens if he takes out a large weed and does not use the weed-killer thereafter. The patient answered proudly that obviously the weeds would grow right back because the roots were still there and that without the weedkiller, the likelihood of remaining weed-free was very low.

The doctor then said to the patient that removing his lung cancer without treating him with the appropriate adjuvant chemotherapy was like pulling out a large weed and not using the weed killer because microscopic cancer cells can be left behind which can lead to recurrence.

Chemotherapy (and other modalities) was one of the ways that we could try to prevent this from happening.

There was a long silence in the room as this patient processed this illustration that now made it make sense to him.

Needless to say, he proceeded with the recommended therapy. This takes extra time but definitely has the benefit of the patient being given the opportunity to feel that he, at least in part, understands the rationale for your recommendation and also helps him in his journey toward acceptance.

Understanding goes a long way in effecting acceptance and action. Understanding, is how you move from compliance with recommendations to adherence to a plan.

Because when the patient understands, he too appreciates (at least in part) the rationale behind the decision, can weigh the risks and benefits for himself, and can take ownership of the decision to proceed (or not), rather than feeling that he is being simply being TOLD what to do.

Some patients prefer a more paternalistic approach, and would rather be told what to do, but I find that these patients state that preference quite clearly, and usually quite early on.

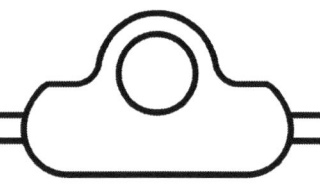

## BOTTOM LINE

Try to speak to patients in a way that they can understand fundamentally.

Provide simple illustrations and analogies that are culturally relatable.

# ℞ ACTION PLAN

- [ ] Think of two common disorders that you treat almost daily. Think of the questions that you commonly get asked.

# ℞ ACTION PLAN

- [ ] Try to think of a simple illustration that you can use to explain to a patient what happens when this disorder occurs or what happens during your proposed therapy to make them feel better. Sometimes it comes to you easily and sometimes it takes some thought...but believe me, when you find it, it's a gold mine in terms of your ability to quickly relate to patients in a way that no one else has in the past. An interaction like that can change your life and the more you practice and tailor it, the better it becomes, and the more you find that you will answer the questions before they are even asked. It shows them that it matters that they understand what is happening.

## CHAPTER 13

# The Power of Navigating Difficult Patient Scenarios Well

Rest assured, difficult scenarios will find you! They come in all shapes, sizes, and variations, and no two situations are exactly the same. The art of working through difficult patient scenes comes with experience, comfort with yourself, sound medical and clinical knowledge that can serve to back you up, and finally, plain old common sense.

While I cannot possibly prepare you for every difficult situation that you will encounter in your practice, I can give you some insight into how I managed to navigate through a few of my own. There are also some hypothetical scenarios that we will review which can help us to walk through how you could possibly manage in a similar situation.

The difficulties and awkward moments that you may encounter will be heavily influenced by your specialty and the specifics of your clinical practice, but general principles of crisis management are likely to hold true.

## *Denying A Patient Request, in Their Best Interest*

Mrs. Black was referred to me by a plastic surgeon for evaluation and management of her uncontrolled diabetes before undergoing cosmetic surgery. She had planned a tummy tuck and butt lift, having recently embarked on a fitness journey after having five children.

Eagerly anticipating her procedure, which was already scheduled for just a few weeks later from her appointment with me, Mrs. Black had already made non-refundable arrangements for travel and accommodation. Her only request from me was a letter deeming her 'sugar levels' satisfactory for surgery.

Despite her anticipation; a detailed history, examination, and an immediate Hemoglobin A1C test revealed her diabetes to be significantly uncontrolled, with an A1C level of 11.2%.

She confidently stated she felt fine and was ready to manage her diabetes rigorously after her surgery. However, as she pressed for the clearance letter, becoming increasingly impatient during our discussion about her condition, I found myself in a professional and ethical quandary.

I had to explain that proceeding with her surgery under such uncontrolled diabetic conditions posed serious risks, including heightened infection rates and other complications that could mar the outcomes she desired.

Despite the potential that things might go smoothly, the risks were too high—risks that both the surgeon and anesthesiologist would likely deem unacceptable as well.

When I voiced my inability to in good conscience provide the clearance she sought, Mrs. Black's frustration boiled over. She tearfully accused me of wasting her time and resources, lamenting, "Thank you for wasting my time. I have spent a lot of time and money to have this procedure, and I don't see why we can't handle this after I return!"

Her departure was as emotional as it was swift, leaving behind a palpable tension and a profound sense of professional duty on my part. While difficult, this scenario underscored the importance of prioritizing patient health over their immediate desires, a principle that occasionally leads to hard, yet necessary decisions.

Despite the pressure and the emotional charge of the moment, my commitment to her best interest remained unwavering—a commitment that often requires difficult conversations and decisions that might not align with a patient's immediate expectations or desires.

## BOTTOM LINE

Do what is best for your patient even when they pressure you to do otherwise.

You can't win every battle.

When things go wrong, often people will point the finger at you! Try to stick to what you know and to what you know that you should do.

# ℞ ACTION PLAN

- [ ] Think of a scenario when you would have to deny a patient something that they request. How would you handle such a scenario?

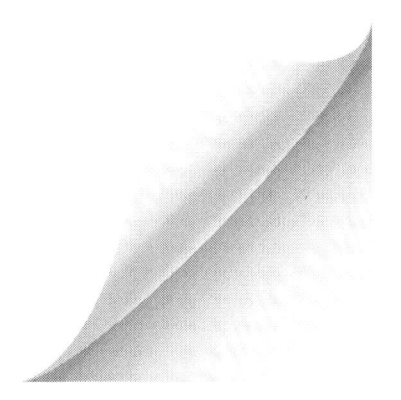

# The Power of Navigating Difficult Patient Scenarios Well

*PART 2: BREAKING BAD NEWS*

In my specialty, I rarely break what is generally considered to be really bad news. I care for patients who have endocrine disorders or chronic medical disorders and rarely are they acutely ill.

The art of breaking bad news, for some, is a difficult one to master. Remaining compassionate and sincere while protecting yourself from emotional burnout is an interesting balance to keep.

### Navigating Timelines and Prognoses

We know of patients receiving catastrophic diagnoses or terminal diagnoses and being told that they have six months to live by their specialist. I would generally recommend that people stay away from giving patients definitive timelines. It is probably ok to say that patients like you in age, sex, diagnosis, and stage of disease would typically survive 'x' months or years with standard therapy. Some will exceed these expectations and others, for various reasons, may not survive as long.

This removes you from being perceived as one who believes himself the all-knowing oracle, as this is typically not well accepted by patients and their families. Try, as much as possible, to go with statistics and generalities and offerings of what is typical. This allows you to simply be a source of information and not a predictor of outcome. This is also true in the opposite scenario, where persons with the condition that your patient was just diagnosed with typically live very long and productive lives.

Resist the temptation to be overly confident with your words and simply state that in patients similar to yourself, there is typically a 95% survival rate at 5 years and that most of my patients, who receive appropriate care without unforeseen complications or other circumstances, far exceed this expectation. You have hereby given facts and hope without directly being one who tries to predict what will happen with any one specific patient at any one particular time. I suppose that it is ok to say that I expect, that if all goes according to plan, you will do just as well.

As we know, in the fraternity of medicine, anything can happen, so try very hard to be objective in your answers and try to remove all emotional connections (positive or negative) when answering such questions of prognosis.

You can be positive and direct, when necessary, but you get the point, be careful with how you allow yourself to predict 'how much time' someone has left. Doing this is laden with risk and problems, even if you are correct.

## *The Importance of Careful Communication*

Imagine giving a patient a diagnosis with a poor prognosis and telling them that he has 4 months to live. You then go on to tell the patient and the family that we can go ahead and 'try' this regimen and see if it helps.

At this point, you have sent a very interesting signal, and there may be a sense of giving up on the patient and doing some pointless regimen that you know won't help.

It is possible that when this patient does in fact die 4 months later, the family is left feeling that you didn't offer the best therapy in the first place because you never truly believed that their relative could live. They walk away feeling that you didn't even try and that you just let their relative die.

Conversely, they may ask why you put their relative through that if you knew it was pointless…they may feel that perhaps you wanted to bill more for unnecessary visits or allow the hospital to bill for therapy that was futile.

So, how you word something is oh so important. Imagine instead telling them that the prognosis in this scenario is typically poor, but that some patients exceed expectations when given the recommended therapy.

You can advise that although a certain expectancy is typical, you would ask them to consider the option of therapeutic intervention to give themselves or their relative the best chance at more time.

You would also take into consideration the potential side effects of the proposed therapy and the impact that it might have on the quality of the remaining life that the patient has, and this would be weighed against the quality of life expected if the patient were to remain untreated.

So, yes, the approach to breaking 'bad news' does warrant some extra thought and preparation and depending on your degree of comfort, some practice too.

## *Addressing Prediabetes and Diabetes*

So, let's talk about the bad news that I do have to break as an endocrinologist. When a patient is referred to me or presents to my office for evaluation and management, I often have the task of informing patients that they are diabetic or pre-diabetic.

In some cases, this was not even the reason for the consultation, but it was noted as an elevation in the fasting glucose or hemoglobin A1C. I often ask the patient if they were advised that their recent labs indicated that they were diabetic (or prediabetic). Often, I am met with shock, surprise, and genuine disbelief.

I would just like to put an endo plug in here and advise that prediabetes is a real thing. It is an actual diagnosis, and it is actionable; but if no intervention is initiated, the majority of these patients will progress to overt diabetes and develop the dreaded complications if not well controlled.

It's not ok to tell them that their sugar was 'A little elevated' and that 'we will just watch it'. Giving them a diagnosis tends to drive home the gravity of the situation and telling someone that their sugar is a little elevated trivializes a rather serious metabolic condition and could cause someone to miss the opportunity to intervene.

If you are uncomfortable giving appropriate advice or you simply don't have the time, then refer the patient to someone who can help. I have even gone as far as to tell patients that they have a disorder that I have coined 'pre-pre-diabetes'.

I of course inform them, that such a diagnosis does not exist (yet). But I tend to go on to explain that if a fasting glucose of 100mg/dl or above gives them a diagnosis of prediabetes then a fasting glucose of around 96-99mg/dl indicates that they are likely on their way to prediabetes if they change nothing about their lifestyle.

So, I tell them that they have, what I have coined 'pre-pre-diabetes' and we begin initiating lifestyle interventions and following their glucose parameters periodically, as we would someone with diabetes or prediabetes.

The same goes for someone with a hemoglobin A1C of 5.6 or 5.5%, where they have not met the criteria for prediabetes, but probably would if they continued with the sedentary and carbohydrate-laden lifestyle choices.

## *Reframing the Diagnosis as an Opportunity*

Often, I would advise patients that finding out they are prediabetic or diabetic is actually good news, especially when this diagnosis is made early on.

I would tell patients that many people in populations like our own are not diagnosed with diabetes or prediabetes when they have an opportunity to intervene with intensive lifestyle therapy and medications if needed, before they develop complications.

I advise them that those who do not undergo regular annual physical exams can go for years with no idea that they are diabetic and that many remain undiagnosed, untreated, and uncontrolled for many years before coming to medical attention.

Further, by the time they do present themselves for care, it is in the context of some metabolic catastrophe, or it is long after they have started to develop complications.

So, I tell my patients that being diagnosed with prediabetes or diabetes early allows them the opportunity that many do not have, to change the outcome of this story and to completely take control and change the narrative.

The typically asymptomatic nature of uncontrolled diabetes and hypertension allows them to wreak havoc internally for years while going unnoticed.

So yes, having access to annual physicals and screenings and diagnosing things early before the onset of complications can be framed as good news, and many patients leave having been empowered to intervene on their own behalf.

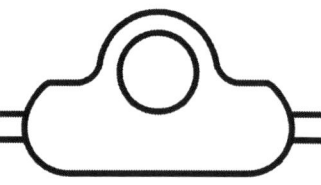

## BOTTOM LINE

You can get better at breaking bad news.

You can practice breaking bad news until you become comfortable doing it.

Some bad news can be framed as good news or as an opportunity to change, depending on the scenario.

## ℞ ACTION PLAN

☐ Think of a scenario where you may have to break bad news, preferably a scenario that you encounter frequently. Practice how you would approach delivering this bad news. Practice out loud and if you are uncomfortable, reach out to someone that you know is more comfortable at delivering bad news and ask them what they think of your approach. You're not bothering them, just tell them that you notice that they are good at handling these situations and you would appreciate a little coaching in that regard.

# ℞ ACTION PLAN

- [ ] Everyone loves being regarded as an expert. They will probably find some time for you. If this is not practical, consider doing an online palliative care course or do some reading online or from a book on breaking bad news. You can also check out videos or other resources that may be on the internet. The whole point is to be intentional about improving yourself in this area if needed.

# The Power of Navigating Difficult Patient Scenarios Well

## *PART 3: TALKING ABOUT SEX*

Talking about sex is an interesting one, and often comes up in my encounters as I often care for patients with chronic medical disorders and also those with hormonal disorders that can affect the sexual act or the reproductive potential or both.

I often find that after a few visits with me, or perhaps at the end of an initial visit, often for another concern, patients would bring up their intimate concerns. They often find creative ways to segue into the topic of difficulty with erections or decreased libido.

The irony is that by virtue of my training at a few VA hospitals, I started my practice more comfortable managing male reproductive concerns than those of females.

The market, and my patient population, have demanded that I become comfortable with the issues faced by both males and females and I am certain, that if I am blessed with a long enough life, my own physiology will demand that I continue to become even more comfortable helping women manage their reproductive lives, especially as it relates to menopause and the myriad of changes that come along with that.

## The Importance of Discussing Sex and Sexuality

The topic of sex is important in so many contexts as medical professionals. As primary physicians, discussing the natural changes that occur as we traverse the life cycle is important. Sex and sexuality as we age, are important topics of discussion and important aspects of life that require addressing.

And yes, it does fall into your purview. Sometimes patients' sexual concerns may stop them from taking medications that may help them in other aspects, and that could have been easily substituted for other medications that may have posed less of a risk of sexual side effects. Sometimes lifestyle changes may have been all that was needed to control an elevated blood pressure or an elevated glucose level.

## Discussing Bodies, Private Parts, and Safety with Children

As pediatricians and family doctors, I imagine interesting conversations as you guide adolescents through the changes in their bodies and as you guide parents with suggestions about how to address these changes and hormonal surges and new desires and impulses.

It is so important that you recognize the need as medical professionals and people caring for young children to discuss the topics surrounding their bodies, their private parts, their sexuality, and their safety very early on, because they have the potential to be exposed to so much so soon!

With access to technology and to people around them, it might be beneficial for you as the doctor or parent to start to have discussions with children about their bodies and to try to create a 'safe zone' where they feel comfortable asking their questions without fear of judgment or reprimand. We want them to get information from us as early as is appropriate (and that will depend on many things), because there are people out there waiting to influence your children.

The proactive intervention will at least allow you the opportunity to start to shape their thinking and their experience so that they have some frame of reference or degree of 'grounding' before being bombarded with the plethora of information, misinformation, and 'choices' that they will be faced with.

I cannot imagine being a young person today, but then I must, because I'm around young people, and if I am to stand even a remote chance of influencing them, I have to be more prepared than I was prepared to be.

## *Addressing Fertility Concerns in Cancer Patients*

As oncologists, you may be faced with patients who have cancers or disorders, the treatment of which, may impair or completely compromise their fertility or sexual function.

You might be a standout by familiarizing yourself, even on the most basic level, with fertility preservation interventions and by finding a favorite fertility clinic in your area to refer your patients to. You may (or may not) be surprised about how many people don't give this a thought until after the fact, when it may be more difficult or in fact too late.

Help your patients, they are dealing with a lot, and they may not even have the presence of mind to consider life as a cancer survivor. They may be too young for fertility to be a consideration at their current life stage. Think for them, they are depending on you in this vulnerable time, and one conversation could spark a life-changing decision.

## *Addressing Sexual Concerns in Cancer Patients*

On another note, your chemotherapy patients may be withholding sex from their partners, or the partners may be afraid to engage in sexual intercourse because of fears about toxicities or side effects from chemotherapy affecting the partner who is not being treated.

These patients may not share these concerns with you and may carry on having compromises in a relationship which is already being challenged by cancer and all that comes with it.

Let's be proactive and spend the extra three minutes bringing up topics that may prolong our visits, but may make a world of difference in the life of a patient by answering a few questions, allaying a few concerns, or dispelling a few myths or misconceptions.

## *The Role of Gynecologists in Female Reproductive Health*

As gynecologists, I would presume that you are very comfortable handling the reproductive concerns of your patients. You are the cornerstone of female health maintenance and restoration. Don't forget to talk about the practical concerns that women may have as they traverse the many stages of life.

And remember, if a couple is trying to conceive for a prolonged period of time, 'more time' is probably not the answer. Refer them to a fertility specialist to discuss their options. I remember being told by a gynecologist once that they do not believe in 'infertility.'

That was diabolical, but did not harm our relationship in any way. I guess they feel that if you try long and hard enough, you'll get pregnant. Perhaps this has been their experience, but for those who may not end up that lucky, please refer them to someone who 'believes' and not only believes, but can help.

## *Addressing Hereditary Concerns*

Many patients want to know if their children are at risk for developing the condition that they have. Most patients, in my experience, would ask this upfront as it does not directly address the sexual act.

So, it might be prudent to briefly brush up on the heritability of the conditions that you treat often. No one is expecting a geneticist's dissertation from you, but they would at least like to know if it is very likely, somewhat likely, or not very likely at all to affect their children. Also, familiarize yourself with recommendations for screening for their conditions in offspring.

## *Addressing Sexual Concerns in Various Medical Specialties*

I suppose I would have to leave it to the orthopedic specialists to discuss sex with patients maintained in traction of the lower extremities, that's beyond my current level of training, experience, and expertise.

But by now, you get what I am saying, your patients have concerns about how their conditions will affect sex and about how sex affects their condition and their partner.

Many patients may be anxious to bring up the topic, so go ahead and think about how sex is likely to be affected by your patient's condition or treatment, and ease the tension by gently bringing up the topic.

If they state that they have no concerns, perhaps think of a few common questions or concerns that have come up with other patients or that you think may be relevant given their current condition, and give a few pointers or words of advice or caution.

Although it may be unsolicited, it will likely be very appreciated now or in the future.

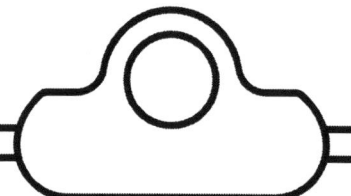

## BOTTOM LINE

Sex is important to many of your patients.

Reproduction and reproductive potential are important to many of your patients.

Many of your patients will be too shy to bring up their sexual concerns with you.

Many of them will 'open up' once you have introduced the topic and have made it ok to talk about it.

# ℞ ACTION PLAN

- [ ] Remember to find a way to ask patients about how their condition may affect their intimacy and also to ask them if they have any concerns about how their condition or treatment will affect their sexual or reproductive health.

- [ ] Do not assume that sex is not a relevant topic to discuss because your patient is an older individual.

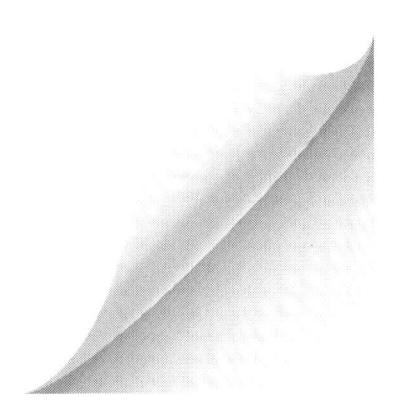

# The Power of Navigating Difficult Patient Scenarios Well

## *Part 4: Fertility Issues*

This topic is so near and dear to my heart because as an endocrinologist, I see many patients with reproductive concerns. Sometimes it is within my realm of expertise to assist them, and sometimes they require even more subspecialized care and interventions.

When taking a history from a patient, I have learned to always tread carefully around the topic of children.

We often take for granted that people who want children just go ahead and have them. Easy peasy, right? It is such a sensitive topic, and in some cases, a very painful one.

I find gentle ways of asking if people have children, especially when it is very relevant to the medical condition. We must remember that subfertility and infertility are very common and can be as frequent as one in four to one in six couples, according to some sources.

So, if you have not had reproductive challenges, chances are that you know someone who has had a challenge, whether or not you are aware of it.

## Cultural Pressures and Insensitive Comments

In Caribbean culture, and perhaps in other cultures, everyone believes that they have a right to other people's reproductive information.

From aunties, grandparents, parents, friends, and cousins, to people in the church and random people in the community, it is quite commonplace for people at a family gathering to look at a couple and make some insensitive proclamation along the lines of, "Y'all been married for five years now, y'all don't think it's time to have children?"

Another question is, "What are y'all waiting for?" I was once told by an aunt, unsolicited I might add, "Well, you better hurry up, you know, you ain't no spring chicken no more!"

Yep, these were words of advice to which I had no response. There was not a man somewhere out there in an envelope just waiting for me to find the envelope opener. What kind of advice is that? I am not even sure how I responded.

I remember another time meeting an elderly distant relative or in-law who, at the dinner table, proclaimed that when she first met me, she felt sorry for my husband because she just knew that I would not be willing to give up my "body" to have any children for him! True story!

I believe that I responded, "Well, I was taught that if I don't have anything nice to say, I must not say anything at all; therefore, I cannot say anything to you!" That was our last conversation. Audacity!

## The Emotional Impact on Patients

Oh, my heart bleeds for my patients. The tears that have been shed in my presence could fill a river and sail a yacht. These comments are so damaging, and people really have no business interjecting themselves into the reproductive adventures or misadventures of a couple, a woman, or a man for that matter.

I know women who dread family gatherings simply because the looks, gazes, and questions are virtually inevitable, and it hurts so much to smile and engage when inside you want to die. They want so badly to say, "Mind your own business!" ... but they won't do it.

## *Insensitivity in the Medical Field*

What saddens me most is the fact that these people are not immune to such judgment when they come to the physician. They would think that the doctor's office is a safe space and that at least a doctor would understand that sometimes medical issues can interfere with reproductive potential and success.

I once referred a patient to another physician for a specialized opinion. She advised me that she would never see that doctor and that I must immediately find someone else because "that doctor is a devil!" Yes, she said those words.

I looked at her, and she proceeded to explain that she had had two miscarriages in the past and had sought a medical opinion from this doctor who looked at her and asked her, "When are you going to stop doing this foolishness? You cannot have a baby!" Those may not have been the exact words, but you get the point.

Now, at the time of our meeting of course, this is the proud mother of a healthy 6-year-old child, and this occurrence was over 8 years prior. Perhaps the doctor was making a valid point; perhaps the patient had a medical condition that made pregnancy improbable or even dangerous for her.

But was this the way to advise her that attempting to carry a baby to term was ill-advised and could be a threat to both her life and her unborn child's life? Clearly not!

## *Treating Patients with Compassion*

As physicians, we must try to remember that patients are just people who have medical conditions. They are not a medical condition, and they are not a disease. They are not a "case" of a 36-year-old female with lupus. She is a woman, a sister, a daughter, and an auntie. She is a student, an accountant, or a singer with hopes, dreams, and ambitions just like you have.

Be sensitive in how you communicate with people. While some things may seem medically obvious to you, this might be an entirely new and unexpected turn of events that causes someone to question their entire existence.

Imagine if it were your sister and some doctor made her cry with unnecessarily harsh words. You would be LIVID! So, step back, and when you find yourself tempted to be callous, take a break and walk away, excuse yourself for a moment, and recompose.

## *The Importance of Referrals and Timely Intervention*

Also, with regards to fertility, this could come under the power of referring, but I will make the point here because it is such an important point. It is absolutely sad to have a couple trying to conceive naturally for a decade without mentioning the possibility of assisted reproductive technologies or without investigating appropriately to see if something organic, tangible, and treatable is making pregnancy difficult. Your moral stance on the matter is irrelevant.

I have met more than a few women, in excess of forty years of age, who are now seeking advice about reproductive potential after being with a physician for many years. After 6 to 12 months of attempting to conceive without success, depending on the age of the couple, they should be referred for evaluation of possible anatomical, hormonal, or other impediments. It's so important to do this before age also becomes a factor in their reproductive journey.

I have spent so much time on this topic because it is a topic that takes up a lot of time in my clinical practice. So, in addition to being sensitive with how you take a reproductive history, remember to remain nonjudgmental and compassionate because every story is so different.

If your patient is trying to conceive, refer them to someone who can help them or at least to someone who knows who to refer them to. Encouraging patients to continue having "faith" without doing the appropriate workup and then "works" can be folly.

## *Caring for Ourselves as Medical Professionals*

As we navigate the process of engagement in our RACE and C.A.R.E. framework, it is a timely place to pause and consider again our engagement with our true selves. Becoming a medical doctor, and further, a medical specialist or subspecialist takes TIME... yes, it takes time, along with all the other things that it takes from us and requires of us.

As we race through the days, the nights, the exams, the applications, the interviews, the calls, and all the other demands that are placed on us, we must remember to pause and consider caring for ourselves.

## *Considering Our Own Reproductive Journey*

For women especially, as we consider the reproductive journey of our patients, we must remember to consider our own. We must ask ourselves the tough questions because we can't table the issues indefinitely.

We must foresee interesting realities that many of us will face. As we become more and more qualified and spend more and more time in school, institutions of higher learning, or in booming careers, the chances of pairing off into a committed long-term relationship or marriage become less and less likely.

This is by no means to suggest that "pairing off" or "getting married" are somehow what every woman is hoping for or even should hope for, but the reality is that many of us do hope for this and hope for the life that we think that it affords.

The second consideration is that the older we get, the less likely are our chances of natural conception, or any conception really. If these things are of importance to you and if you have not considered them before, it may be time to take pause and consider your options. Should you make more time for dating?

Should you be considering the fact that single people in your "circle" could be potential mates? Should you have taken a proposition a little more seriously and not shrugged it off, assuming that there will always be more, or that you can revisit it when you have more time? Should you be considering assisted reproductive technologies and fertility preservation techniques?

Many of the hospitals that we rotate through as medical students, residents, and fellows have thriving reproductive endocrinology practices or are affiliated with them. If not, there may be one nearby if you are in a major city.

Some of us will even do rotations at fertility clinics depending on our specialties and would never consider the option for ourselves, because we are so focused on academia and the need to get through it. Consider these things if you are single or in a relationship or even married and feel that the time is just not quite right.

These are conversations that no one has with us as we grow up and that we perhaps wish they did. These are the things in your quiet times that you contemplate and ruminate over and start to wonder, "What if?"

## *Seeking Help When Needed*

As you matriculate through your extensive academic and professional journey, you must be reminded to consider your reproductive and other needs and desires, as by the time the dust settles, it may be too late. Now, if you find yourself at the peak of success's mountain but upon introspection you find that you are actually in an emotional valley, for any reason, then seek help!

You may need emotional help, physical help, spiritual help, medical help, or all of the above. Reach out and seek the help that you need. You cannot continue to serve others to the best of your ability if you are nursing secret (or open) wounds that will often betray you.

Love yourself and be true to yourself. It is ok for you to be broken and to recognize it and to seek to repair it. You are not invincible, and needing help does not somehow make you inadequate... but it most certainly makes you human.

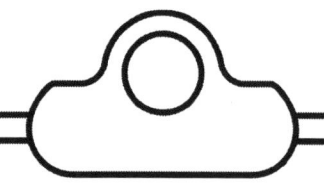

> **BOTTOM LINE**
>
> Many patients suffer in silence and fail to mention their concerns for fear of judgment or insensitive comments or questions.
>
> Many doctors do the same.

# Rx ACTION PLAN

- [ ] If you are a doctor, be sensitive and gentle in how you take a reproductive history.

- [ ] If a medical condition makes childbearing dangerous for a patient, you can advise them of this quite firmly, but you can also be sensitive in your approach.

- [ ] Reproduction can affect many conditions and many conditions can have effects on reproductive journeys, don't forget to ask about it as you treat your patient.

# ℞ ACTION PLAN

- [ ] If you come across a man or woman or couple that is childless, be careful, you do not know what is really going on and one callous or ill-considered comment can have supremely negative effects. Think before you speak.

- [ ] If your own reproductive potential is something that you have never considered, think about having a conversation with your gynecologist.

## CHAPTER 14

# The Power of Serving as The Doctor to A Doctor

There is a special group of physicians who will be called upon to serve as the physician for another medical doctor. While this is indeed a special honor, privilege, and pleasure, it certainly is a challenge and brings with it special nuances that are not present in other physician-patient relationships.

While being chosen by a colleague can make one feel as though they were specially selected by someone with specialized knowledge, there is a pressure that comes along with this duty. Doctoring a doctor can be quite intimidating and it is important to remember to just be yourself and do your job.

You must acknowledge and accept that being a doctor to a physician comes with many pressures, some often self-imposed. Namely, a pressure to do well, a pressure not to miss anything, a pressure to get it right, and a pressure not to mess anything up. While this pressure is present in any physician's relationship with a patient, it is magnified, in my experience, when caring for a colleague or fellow physician.

Navigating this relationship requires a certain degree of intentionality and demands that you be aware of some of the pitfalls that can complicate the interactions.

We must be guarded against assumptions that we make when we are talking to our physician-patient. As I have had both the pleasure and the challenge of being on both sides of this equation, I have had the opportunity to both witness many missteps, and also the distinct pleasure of making them.

Each time that I am given the opportunity to serve a physician-patient in this capacity, I am able to refine my skill in playing this role even more. We will explore a few cautionary steps that you ought to always be aware of.

### *Treat Your Physician-Patient as a Patient, Not a Colleague*

Firstly, don't fall into the trap of treating your physician-patient as a physician or colleague. He or she is a patient and simply a patient. DO NOT cut to the chase. Do not assume that they know what is relevant to their presenting complaint and that therefore would tell you all of the relevant information up front.

This can cause you to remain focused only on the complaint, therefore bypassing some information in the history. You may miss an important detail that may have materially redirected your decision-making process. You might make the wrong decision.

Introduce yourself to the patient, thank them for seeking your services as a physician, and advise them that you will be taking the usual course of management as you would with any other patient. Then, get started. Take a full history, and do a complete physical examination just as you would in the course of any other patient interaction.

### *Use Plain Language and Avoid Assumptions*

To take this further, once you have done your history and exam and you have decided on a differential diagnosis, or even if the diagnosis is pretty clear to you, discuss with your patient exactly what you think is going on in plain and simple terms.

Commonly used medical jargon can be ok but be careful not to use super specialized terminology with your patient. It is probably safer just to explain things in plain language as we discussed earlier in this book. This protects both of you from precarious situations.

For instance, you might tell this patient that after your history, examination, and review of his labs, you think he may have cholelithiasis and that he should have a right upper quadrant ultrasound and after you review the results at the follow-up visit, he may need to be referred to a gastroenterologist or to a surgeon for further management.

You make several assumptions when you speak to your physician-patient in this way. You assume that he or she knows what cholelithiasis is. He may be too embarrassed to tell you that he doesn't and may simply smile and nod and go along with what you are saying.

He may not want to be seen as a doctor who doesn't even know what cholelithiasis is. He may be so far removed from the general knowledge of medical school and so deeply enshrined in his specialty for the past 25 years that the meaning of this word may have escaped him.

The other scenario is that he is like me and would say, 'What is cholelithiasis' and you look at him as if he is a complete moron who obviously never paid attention in medical school and should be ashamed to not know what that is. There we created an awkward moment that could hurt this relationship. On the other hand, you could handle his question like a champ.

But how about you avoid all of this in the first place by saying, 'I think you may have gallstones and I recommend that we do an ultrasound of your liver and gallbladder!' This was simple, and avoided any chance of letting assumptions interfere with your relationship. So, keep it simple doc!

## Be Cautious of Self-Diagnoses

Be very aware when the physician-patient comes to you with a self-diagnosis. While your colleague may be an excellent and knowledgeable physician, remember to stick with the first principles. Take a history, do a physical examination, and proceed with your confirmatory investigations as appropriate. Follow the algorithm. It generally works.

I remember the story of a patient coming to a colleague some years ago to treat her menopause. She was having hot flashes and mood swings and was irritable and had difficulty sleeping. She was about 52 years old and had a last period about 16 months prior. She was clearly in menopause and had done her labs to prove it and wanted to explore the possibility of hormone replacement therapy.

She wanted to get right to the point and discuss the risks and benefits of hormone replacement therapy in herself as she had no personal or family history of breast cancer or ovarian cancer and she is a nonsmoker with no personal or family history of heart disease or blood clots. Her heat intolerance and irritability were interfering with her job and her family, and she was ready to get her prescription, to get her medication, and to feel better and close this chapter!

The endocrinologist was also convinced of her new patient's diagnosis but explained that she would just like to do a routine history and physical exam. The physician-patient was quite unexcited to agree as she runs a busy practice and didn't want to prolong this visit with the 'unnecessaries' given that she had a clear-cut diagnosis and she had already brought the lab results with her.

Reluctantly, she agreed to allow her doctor to proceed. Turns out she was 4 years behind on her annual physical exams, and had no colonoscopy and no mammogram or pap smear for about that amount of time. Her response was that she was low-risk and busy and that she was fine and would get around to it at some point. On exam, the endocrinologist noticed a fine tremor and that her reflexes were a little hyperreactive.

Finally, she was also noted to have a mildly enlarged thyroid gland. The doctor looked at her patient and said to her, while you may be menopausal, I believe that your symptoms may actually be due to thyrotoxicosis, if not in whole, at least in part. I'm going to send you for routine lab testing including thyroid function tests and I am going to refer you for a pap smear and mammogram to complete your annual physical exam. I will see you in a few days to review your results. She decided to do her labs the following morning and was seen the next day as her labs revealed thyrotoxicosis.

Treatment for her hyperthyroidism was immediately initiated and the patient was seen for clinical follow-up in about two weeks and most of her symptoms had subsided or improved. The mammogram and pap smear were planned with a family physician for the following week. The colonoscopy was to be planned once the thyrotoxicosis was well managed.

This patient presented herself with symptoms and labs to support her diagnosis and was insistent on being treated. While hyperthyroidism is rarely life-threatening, untreated thyrotoxicosis can lead to severe and even fatal complications. This patient was appropriately managed because her doctor insisted on following protocol and resisted the pressure to treat her colleague outside of the parameters of a traditional physician-patient relationship.

No one would have understood how she went to an endocrinologist who missed a clear diagnosis of hyperthyroidism in a patient who had heat intolerance, emotional lability, and difficulty sleeping. She also had a fine tremor and some weight loss that she didn't mention. No one would have been there to see the interaction, but they would hear about her ending up in hospital with thyroid storm after being treated for menopause by an endocrinologist who was supposed to be the hormone specialist.

Be very careful and remember that your physician-patient is a patient first. Treat them as such! They will thank you later as this patient eventually did. They addressed the need for hormone replacement therapy after she was rendered euthyroid (after her thyroid hormones normalized) and she decided not to pursue hormone replacement therapy after all.

Remember: history, physical exam, assessment, plan, and ancillary testing. Stick with the protocol, even when your patient is a doctor.

## *Avoid Writing Random Prescriptions*

There is another scenario that can put you in quite a sticky position. It is somewhat like the scenario that we discussed above. This is where a colleague, or someone in general, asks you for a prescription. It seems so benign. In certain practice scenarios, this is not permissible and therefore would not be an issue for certain readers but for others, it is quite commonplace.

This will in most cases proceed without mishap. But it is loaded with risks and should be avoided completely, if possible. I suppose this can be quite awkward if the physician is a close friend, because how do you tell someone that you know and trust 'no'? This can compromise the relationship or at the very least it can create an awkward moment. Perhaps a statement like 'I don't really feel comfortable writing prescriptions for people who are not my patients' might help.

This might require some more thought but if you find this is commonplace and you are not comfortable doing it, you might want to rehearse your response in advance.

On an unrelated topic, this scenario can come up when you are the physician and family members ask for prescriptions. This can happen as a text message, as a phone call, in person at a family gathering, or in other scenarios. They do not understand sometimes what a compromising situation this is for you.

Some physicians have no problem doing it at all, and that is fine, but I am not one of those physicians. I like to keep my relationships clean. I don't know their allergies, their medical conditions, or what other medications they may be taking. Quite frankly, I don't want to take a medical history at the easter egg hunt or at Mother's Day brunch.

Where am I even documenting this encounter? Is this an encounter? Am I now their doctor? I also accept that I may just be a little paranoid, but let's press on.

Suppose she has ulcers and I give her a powerful NSAID for her arthritic knee. Suppose she has an extremely elevated creatinine and I do the same. It can make you feel so mean to say no, but sometimes 'no' is necessary. Your name will be the first name that they call when something goes awry. I try to remain within my comfort zone and writing random prescriptions is not in it. Some may regard me as overly cautious or 'anal' but I like my sleep and I typically try to avoid scenarios that would cause me to lose any of it!

I am not saying that I have not succumbed to this pressure on at least one prior occasion, but I feel more equipped now to say 'no' should the scenario arise again.

## *Caring for the Physician-Patient in the Hospital Setting*

So, that was a long aside, but let us get back to the meat of the matter of caring for the physician who presents himself to you as a patient. Let's discuss the physician-patient for whom you are caring in the hospital setting.

Here is another story of a doctor who took care of another doctor many, many years ago. This patient presented herself to her colleague with a history of right upper quadrant pain. She did have a positive Murphy's sign (tenderness on pressing over the approximate location of the gallbladder) and would have intermittent right upper quadrant abdominal pain when she ate fatty meals and also at other times.

She was overweight and of reproductive age. She was the typical patient that the textbook told us would have gallstones. She had intermittent symptoms that were increasing in frequency and also in intensity to the point where it was a significant bother to her. She had done an ultrasound and also the labs and presented to the surgeon for evaluation for laparoscopic cholecystectomy.

Many physicians (who present to you as patients) do their own investigations. Access allows them to make many decisions and influence many decisions also. She met the surgical criteria, and the procedure was booked. She was scheduled to have a laparoscopic cholecystectomy the following week. The procedure proved to be more challenging than expected because the surgeon began to encounter more and more adhesions that she did not anticipate.

The ease with which the instruments could manipulate the abdominal contents was somewhat restricted. She did lyse some of the adhesions and with some difficulty was eventually able to perform the procedure as planned. When the patient awakened from anesthesia and was doing well in recovery, the surgeon came over to tell her how her procedure went and to let her know that she did have some challenges but that she was able to perform the procedure as planned.

Thankfully she didn't have to convert to an open procedure. The patient then revealed that she had a long history of endometriosis which had been extremely challenging for her to control. This likely contributed to the surgeons' unanticipated difficulties. Recurrent episodes of gallbladder inflammation could also produce more localized adhesions. Fortunately, the procedure went well and both the physician and physician-patient were pleased.

In the end, if she had taken a full history of her patient and examined her, it is very likely that she would have ascertained at some point in that process, that the patient had a risk factor for difficulties during a laparoscopic procedure. She may have been better prepared or may not have offered laparoscopic intervention in the first place.

## *Caring for Your Own Financial Health and Wellness*

As we explored the nuances of serving as a doctor to a doctor and navigated some of the potential pitfalls, this seems like a reasonable time to recommend that we avoid serving as a doctor to ourselves.

Although we touched on this in previous chapters with regards to self-care, listening to your body, and seeking help when appropriate rather than playing superwoman (or superman), we should recognize that in the same way that we need doctors to help us manage our health and trainers to help us to manage our fitness, we also need financial advisers to assist in managing our financial health and wellness.

In the trenches of doctoring, we will find that most of us will make a decent living. Some will become wealthy and some will simply do well. We must remember that we will not be young and able-bodied forever. It is so easy to become caught up in the moment and to just live and enjoy the few moments that we get to enjoy.

We work, we pay bills, we pay taxes, we pay fees, we take vacations, and we do many other things. Remember to plan for your future. Remember to put a portion of your income aside that will be sufficient to help sustain you in your retirement years.

It seems so weird to have to say this but many physicians find themselves in a state of poor financial health. We generally don't receive formal financial training and many of us can be naïve when it comes to wealth planning, estate planning, appropriate insurance, and appropriate savings and investment plans. I know many physicians working well after their expected retirement age.

Some of this may be because of sheer love of medicine, some because they do not know what they would do if they stopped practicing, and some are working to sustain themselves even though they had a thriving medical career and probably had significant amounts of money pass through their fingers. Although we are generally regarded as, and usually are highly intelligent, we must learn to recognize the areas of knowledge deficiencies and address them appropriately and in a timely manner.

It would be remiss if I were to give you advice about how to develop yourself as an excellent physician communicator and practitioner and to lead you beyond the knowledge, if I did not also advise you to remember to care for your medical, spiritual, mental, psychological, physical, sexual, emotional, and financial health.

You are a whole person and to be whole you must acknowledge all the dimensions of your health and address them. Remember that although you are the one who is sought after for help, you will at times need to seek help.

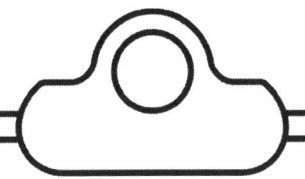

## BOTTOM LINE

The physician-patient is a patient! Beware not to accept self-diagnoses prematurely.

Physicians can misdiagnose themselves. Follow the process. It generally works.

Take a full history and examine your patient, even if she or he is a doctor themselves.

# R<sub>x</sub> ACTION PLAN

- [ ] If you have the privilege and challenge of doctoring a doctor, do your best to treat that patient as you would any other patient in terms of your diagnostic and management process. Yes, physician courtesies will exist, but don't let them compromise your judgment and decision-making.

- [ ] If you are currently doctoring yourself, reconsider this.

- [ ] Seek help for yourself in the dimensions where you are not capable of excellence.

# CHAPTER 15

# The Power of Caring for the Patient Whose Close Family Member is A Physician

Closely related to the challenge of caring for a physician as a patient, is the scenario of caring for the patient whose relative is a physician. It may be that the physician brought the relative to you, recommended you, or knows you personally and recommended that their spouse, parent, child, or other relative come to see you for a concern. Sometimes you discover that there is a physician in the family later on.

In general, this is not a problem. It can create more work sometimes when physician-relatives demand exhaustive explanations and dissertations, but generally, it's ok.

I have had a few pleasant experiences with physician-relatives. I remember having a patient whose sister was a physician. She wanted the discussions to be had with her sister first and then the decision shared with her. Those interactions generally consisted of her presenting to follow-up meetings and calling her sister.

I would review the results and give the guideline-based recommendations. Her sister was not in my field but had done some reading and was quite happy to share that she was not the specialist and that she would defer decisions to me.

My patient simply found comfort in me discussing the plans with her sister, who only asked a few appropriate questions and was generally quite brief and agreeable.

## *When Physician Relatives Overstep Boundaries*

The scenario can get very sticky when physician relatives try to be more involved in the care than is appropriate. This is also quite an interesting interaction when the physician's relative is a colleague.

I do recall treating a patient who had a brother who was a physician. There would be times when I would visit the room to discuss the progress and also the plan with the patient.

Coming to the room sometimes was a complete chore because the brother would make recommendations and also try to decline having certain tests done, claiming that the condition was well within his field of expertise and that the tests were low yield and not likely to reveal any clinically useful information.

The bottom line is that when a patient comes in with certain diagnoses, it is generally recommended that certain baseline tests be done and if this patient were seen at another institution for the condition, the first thing they would look for would be the results of these tests.

They would then proceed to say, 'Wow, what kind of specialist treats a patient with this disorder and does not even get the routine diagnostic testing and secondary testing to rule out the obvious differential diagnoses?'

I now have pressure to act medically appropriately but also pressure to take into consideration what my colleague is saying.

So, I am handling this by politely looking at my colleague and the patient and calmly saying that I will proceed with guideline, clinical, and common sense-directed decision making and I will ask that he play the role of brother in this case.

I advised that judgment can be particularly clouded when emotions are involved and that it is best that he leaves the medical care of his sister to the admitting and consulting physicians. I will be happy to discuss the plan with him and to field questions, but the medical management will be guided by me.

I went on to say that when we are dealing with family, sometimes we want to do too much, and other times we can be dismissive and do too little, taking for granted that 'they will be fine'.

This scenario was very delicate, but with the art of remaining calm and rational, I was able to navigate the waters of putting my physician colleague in his rightful place of being a caring and concerned brother.

Part of me feels that he appreciated that some of his self-induced pressure was publicly taken away from him. Perhaps he felt pressure to perform and to do something to actively improve his sister's situation.

Perhaps he felt that if he said nothing, he would appear helpless and uninvolved in the eyes of his sister. But what his sister needed was her brother. She had lots of physicians and did not need another one at that time.

## *The Pressure to Perform*

Caring for a physician's family member can be challenging in other ways. Sometimes the self-induced pressure to perform is yours. Sometimes the physician knows the prognosis and is quite comfortable with the process that is happening, and you have to resist the temptation to feel the need to perform every test.

This can be especially true in cases where you practice in a small community, and you know many of your colleagues. It is important to remain calm and, for the most part, to act as you would with any other patient.

## *Reserving Judgment*

Also present when treating relatives of physicians, is the need to reserve judgment in scenarios where you feel that this particular matter should have been looked into long before now.

Sometimes we see conditions that are well advanced or that have been lingering long prior to the visit.

In the history, we can be tempted to say things like 'You didn't notice that she was losing height?', or 'Didn't she tell you that the doctor said that her calcium was elevated?', or 'Didn't you notice that she was losing weight?' 'Why did you wait until now to bring her?'

This can add serious insult to injury because you often have no idea what is really going on. You don't know how often this doctor sees his or her parent, and you don't know what it took to get them there.

Perhaps they did notice and had been trying to convince the parent to come in for months and even years. Perhaps they did not know. Perhaps the parent had been keeping the symptoms or the results a secret for any number of reasons.

Perhaps the parent in question is a caregiver to the other parent who is actively ailing, and everyone, including the now patient, spent all their energy and attention on the ill parent while the caregiver parent (now your patient) simply deteriorated.

Just take the history, do the exam, order your investigations, and present the plan of action. This is the safest way to navigate this, and when personal details about the relationship between the two come out, provide nonjudgmental reassurance and encouragement.

## *Respecting Patient Autonomy*

I remember taking care of a patient who had an elevated calcium level. It had been elevated for years and the patient met the criteria for parathyroidectomy for her primary hyperparathyroidism. She was sent to me by her son who was a doctor.

While I tried to convince her that surgical intervention was the way to go, she vehemently refused and we ended up using a bisphosphonate to control hypercalcemia.

Yes, she is a parent to a doctor! Yes, she is hypercalcemic and yes, she is a surgical candidate! However, she is an autonomous, independent individual who is fully capable of making her own decisions.

She made her well-informed decision, and I managed her within the confines of her decision. This has nothing to do with her son, the doctor.

So, while the temptation is to try to coerce her by teaming up with her son, she politely advised that she is the patient and that she will make the decisions as to what is happening with her body.

And guess what, she is right! And her medical care should not be discussed with her son without her expressed permission, so take that! While she did not decide to withhold information from him, she did decide to decline surgical intervention.

Don't forget that the patient is the patient.

## BOTTOM LINE

When doctoring a physician's relative, don't forget who your duties lie with, they lie with the patient.

When doctoring a physician's relative, remember just to follow your routine, it generally works.

When doctoring a physician's relative, remember that you are the doctor and that they are the relative. Sometimes you will have to remind yourself of this fact, and sometimes you will have to remind them of this fact.

# ℞ ACTION PLAN

- [ ] Practice ways to remind a physician that they are the relative and that you are the doctor. This may not always be necessary, but your gut will tell you when it is. If you become comfortable with the idea of doing it, it will come naturally, and you will find your style without being rude or abrasive. It might be necessary to practice it out loud.

- [ ] When doctoring a physician's relative, if this is new to you, step back mentally and remember that this is a patient like anyone else; follow the algorithm, make sound decisions, and remain calm and confident. You are more than capable.

# Chapter 16

# The Power of Doctoring in The Age of Telemedicine

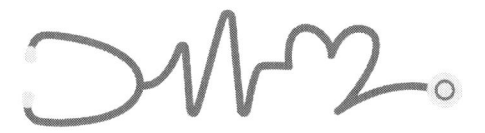

There have been changes to the way we live since 2020. Many of these changes are probably permanent and have influenced us in more ways than we realize. The physical distance between us is now closing, but there are some things that will remain.

It is quite difficult to talk about the power of doctoring, in this day and age, without at least briefly touching on the power of doctoring in the era of telemedicine.

The power of remote physician and health care visits is profound, and has allowed access to care and to specialists to those who would not otherwise have had such access.

In recent history, isolation, quarantine, and social distancing protocols have caused a paradigm shift that touched each of us. In the practice of medicine, there was a gradual acceptance of, and an increase in the use of telecommunication devices to conduct patient care.

## *Challenges and Limitations*

I have had the opportunity to be both the care provider and the care recipient, and both the patient and doctor's experiences are quite different from those to which we are accustomed.

There are many questions and challenges that arise when conducting medicine in this manner. Despite the obvious benefit of access to medical advice when one may not be able to travel to the provider, we must acknowledge the many limitations.

One of my concerns is, how I maintain my personal touch when my patient is being visualized on a device or being interviewed on the telephone.

## *Maintaining Effective Connections*

Thus far, we have talked about the many ways in which to make more effective connections with our patients. Many of the tools that we explored are more easily adapted to a patient being physically present with us.

When having a patient encounter via telemedicine, we must try to be mindful of the many distractors and detractors that can present themselves. Eye contact, for instance, is of paramount importance. It is one of the only visible ways that the patient is assured that they have your attention (when there is a visual component).

Try not to have the cell phone or other device next to you as it is really easy to see when someone's gaze is directed elsewhere. This can make a patient feel that you are paying attention to something else, or worse, that someone else is present in the room where you are conducting the visit, and that their private health information is not so private.

Please be sure that both you and the patient are alone in the encounter, or if the patient is accompanied, that they acknowledge the presence of the other person(s), and that at some point they are visible to you. If you are accompanied by necessary support staff, then acknowledge this also.

## Active Listening and Observation

On the telephone, and on video calls, affirming sounds and nods can add assurance that what the patient is saying is not being lost. They can also force you to listen attentively when there may be a temptation to multitask.

Try to pay attention to body language, facial expressions, pauses, and voice intonations as your physical examination will be limited to observation. Obviously, telemedicine will pose more of a challenge to some specialties than others, but for the most part, the history-taking process would be relatively unscathed.

## The Growing Trend of Telemedicine

Telemedicine was certainly around prior to the social distancing mandates brought about by our experience of 2020 to now, but in my experience, this mode of clinical encounter is becoming more and more commonly offered, and this is a trend not likely to slow down.

Working at being good at telemedicine encounters is worth it in the long run if you are likely to have this as a significant part of your practice. Be mindful of camera positioning and of the lighting in the space where you are.

A camera placed at face and eye level definitely gives a more wholesome and comfortable visual than does one giving the patient a direct line of vision up your nostrils. Poor lighting causes someone to focus on trying to actually see you, versus paying attention to what you are saying.

Be aware of the background where you are. If you are unfamiliar with the space from which you are conducting the encounter, take a quick look behind you or just turn the camera on to see what you look like and what the background looks like before the encounter.

Avoid having too many distracting objects in the line of view. You can also consider using a digital background. This tends to be less of an issue when the interview is conducted from the office, but still, remember to take a quick look.

Remember to smile when it is appropriate to do so. Making natural hand gestures and head nods are other tools to allow you to be physically engaged in the listening process.

## *Addressing Patient Concerns and Understanding*

You can make reference to body language changes if you observe them, and you can bring it up for discussion. It's okay to say to a patient, "I see that this is bothering you, I know that this is a lot to deal with but we will do our best to give you the tools to get through it."

This might be instead of a gentle hand on the shoulder, that might happen if you were in the same room as the patient. You could also say, "Let me put this another way..." if you see that your patient is not understanding what you are saying.

## *Patience with Technological Challenges*

Don't be impatient with technological challenges. These things will happen and as a patient, it's terrifying to think that if there is a disconnection, you would not be able to get back on the call with the doctor.

If the technology fails, ask your staff to assist with reconnecting to the patient. Don't count the encounter as being done.

I remember waiting weeks to have a consultation, and when the consultation began, I was having connection issues. Eventually, I wound up outside the building on my cellphone because I was petrified that if I had lost the connection, I would not get back on the call and that I would have to make another appointment.

I know from experience how busy people can be. I did eventually lose the connection and when I logged back into the virtual waiting room, the doctor was there waiting for me.

When I expressed how grateful I was that he had waited for me to reconnect and how anxious I was that he would be gone, he was quite taken aback. So, remember to be prepared to exercise a little patience as technical difficulties may pose challenges.

Within reason, allow a few minutes for errors, because sometimes the disconnect can be on the part of the provider.

## Controlling Your Environment

Make a special effort to control your environment. Advise family and staff members or other people present in the immediate vicinity that you are about to do a telemedicine call.

If you are at home or in a home office, try to avoid the almost inevitable event of someone inappropriately dressed or undressed making an unannounced entrance into your area. Try to avoid staff walking into the office making announcements or knocking on the door during this protected time.

I remember doing a Zoom meeting when my daughter walked into the room, pulled up her shirt, and started to disrobe herself while announcing that she had to pee. Of course, when you are four years old, it's cute. But it quickly becomes a disturbance if it is frequent.

I remember another instance of being on speaker phone with someone at the lab when a staff member walked in and started announcing that the patient who was supposed to be here 15 minutes ago was now 30 minutes away, she wanted to know what I was going to do and if I was still going to be able to see the patient.

She laughed out loud because she knew how desperately I wanted to leave early that day. She went on to say while laughing vehemently, "So what are you going to do Dr. Parker?" When she finally stopped laughing to see what my response would be, I pointed at the phone and said, "I'm on a call!"

Silence...was the response and she turned away and walked out quickly, apologizing very quietly.

Luckily, no private information was revealed, and her deportment was not egregious, and what she said was not really rude or inappropriate. It was quite typical of our friendly interactions, and she was simply tickled by the irony of my last patient being late on the day that I was trying to leave early.

But just like that, someone has an inside view of what really goes on behind closed doors at your office. It is so important to remain professional at all times, and now I'll get a sign or at least a sticky note indicating when I am on a call.

Yes, I saw the patient. Yes, I stayed late, but luckily, I knew the patient well and there was not much changing. That was a bit off course, but so important. So, let's get back to it.

## *Dressing Appropriately for Telemedicine Encounters*

When working from home, get fully dressed for the encounter. Wearing a shirt and tie and underpants is inappropriate and quite risky as accidents and emergencies do happen and in the thick of the moment, when responding to something, remembering to disable the camera is not likely to actually happen.

We've all seen that commercial on TV with the person at the meeting in the underpants who gets up while the camera is on. While it is undeniably hilarious, your patient does not want to see your underwear or worse.

This type of mishap can negatively affect a physician-patient relationship and is just plain silly and unnecessary.

## *Adapting to Change*

None of us were taught to practice medicine via telehealth visits, this is all relatively new territory for anyone who graduated from medical school more than a few years ago, so we have to make a conscious effort to hone our skills when it comes to this.

I personally prefer in-person encounters, but my preferences will not change the reality of our world in this regard. So, level up and lean into the change. Work on yourself if you find it challenging.

I'm most certain that there is information "out there" on how to conduct a successful virtual interview. You can adapt this to your scenario and take the pearls that work for you and implement them as you see fit.

Also, there are people, probably whom you know, that do it well. Observe them and reach out to them where possible. In the world of change, it is imperative that we adjust and adapt or we will be left behind.

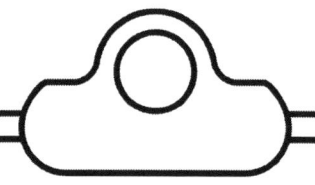

## BOTTOM LINE

You can have impactful virtual patient encounters online.

You can become comfortable with virtual patient encounters where they are appropriate and necessary.

You can adapt to the changing environment and remain relevant in an ever-evolving world.

# ℞ ACTION PLAN

- [ ] Remember to dress fully when holding virtual meetings from home.

- [ ] Remember to organize your background when doing virtual calls and videos from home.

- [ ] When doing a virtual meeting, consider placing a sign or note on the door that you are 'In a Meeting'.

# CHAPTER 17

# The Power of Doctoring in The Age of Artificial Intelligence

Of course, the first person to ask me how I felt about artificial intelligence was a patient. I think that I might have misheard him, or perhaps I wasn't sure what I had heard. He had asked what I thought about 'chat' something and I smiled, but obviously had no clue what he was talking about.

So, of course, he proceeded to tell me about this technology that I was able to ask questions directly to it, and it would just generate the answer. When I was done with my education, and we had concluded the visit, I went to the room with the medical assistants and asked them if they had heard of such a thing... and one of them, of course, whipped out her cellphone and proceeded to ask the app to write her an essay on something...and I watched in awe as the essay was delivered to her screen.

Of course, needless to say, this has been everywhere in the media and I, living in my closed circuit of home, work, church, family, writing, and bed, had managed to completely miss the memo.

I had initially wondered if he had lost confidence in me because I had not heard of the latest tech in A.I., but he did eventually show up again for a follow-up visit. So, if we think about it, the thought of a computer answering medical questions super accurately and helping people can be a bit intimidating.

It can make you question your role as a physician and may even make you wonder if one day you will be obsolete.

## *A Futuristic Vision*

At this point, I am envisioning a kiosk in the mall where I would insert my finger for 6 seconds and perhaps go into the booth and urinate or sweat onto an indicator strip and await the digital transfer or printed output of my diagnosis and treatment plan.

I would then go to the medicine dispenser and insert my credit card or subcutaneously implanted chip and pick up my medications from the dispenser. Or perhaps, I would get dispensed a patch that I can apply and refill weekly or monthly. I might even get an injection in the booth.

I mean, who needs a history and a physical examination anyway?

## *The Presence of AI in Healthcare*

But if we are completely honest with ourselves, we would realize that artificial intelligence has been here for decades, and we have welcomed each and every step in its development to this point.

Who didn't dream of having a Palm Pilot? I believe that we will continue to celebrate its advances as we also remain aware and cautious of the potential challenges that it brings along with it.

At this point, people are wearing watches that collect physiological data and generate reports that patients and physicians can use. Just last week, a patient asked me if I had heard of pulse variability because she had noticed that hers had changed…well, her watch had noticed it.

The amount of information is boundless and there is no way that I can know everything about everything, even in my limited field of specialization, regardless of how much reading I continue to do and how many CME's or conferences I complete.

## *The Burden of Information*

We have used databases to search for information, and patients plug in symptoms into search engines and come to visits with printouts of differential diagnoses and other information to discuss.

The burden of information can also be intimidating, and sometimes you will find that patients know more than you do on a particular esoteric subject, either because they have the condition, think they could have the condition, or are simply interested in it.

I have no problem telling patients that I am not familiar with things, and I am also quite comfortable doing a quick search if I have the time and if I think that it could be relevant to my decision. They are only reading about themselves…you, on the other hand, are reading about all of them.

## *Embracing AI as a Tool*

So, if there is a database out there that takes a record of every single study on a particular disorder or subject and can cross-reference and come up with useful information to help me in seconds, then I choose to see this as a plus.

If there is software that can analyze millions of biopsy results and other analytical calculations and advise the practitioner of the best chemotherapy regimen and biologic or immunologic therapy that is recommended for this individual patient, then let's go.

We will integrate this into our practice and perhaps get information on which side effects are more likely in one person versus another and be able to mitigate the effects. The potential is immense.

## *The Human Touch*

So where do I, as the physician, fit into all this? Well, I do believe that artificial intelligence can outperform me on any exam that requires recall and assimilation of information.

The machine has a potentially unlimited capacity to store and analyze information, I cannot compete with that, and I am a (self-proclaimed) master test taker. Most physicians are. We have had to excel on an immeasurable number of tests to get here, and if we remain board-certified, we are taking exams for our entire careers.

But, for now, at least, I am more than certain that I can outperform any machine, be it intelligent or unintelligent, at being human. I can sit in a room and look at you and know exactly when you need a hug.

And, yes, given the nonverbal and verbal cues, and the physiological changes that I have read can be completely and almost instantaneously analyzed by AI, probably much faster and more accurately than I can, to date, the artificially intelligent machine cannot actually execute the hug, or the therapeutic touch, at least not yet!

The day is probably coming when your nurse or doctor robot will be able to do all of the above. But I maintain that this machine cannot relate to you, and it does not know your cousin or sister.

It is not sharing a common human experience with you and while it may be able to express words of empathy, it will never truly empathize with you, and it will never have a sister or a cousin who went through the exact same thing.

It will never know the exact words to say to you at the exact right time because you are secretly fighting the same battle that your patient is. It will never know what it is like to lose a baby or child or loved one. It will never know what it's like to watch a friend take her last breath.

## *The Unspoken Connection*

When treating patients, there is an unspoken connection that makes a patient connect with one physician over another.

This connection can be because of similar backgrounds, because of similar personalities, because of the person who recommended a particular doctor, because of the development of trust over the course of the relationship, because of the perceived or actual intelligence of the doctor, because of the patient experience, because of the proximity of the doctor and sometimes there is simply a spiritual connection.

While your AI provider can pray at you, probably in any conceivable religion and language, it cannot pray WITH you. I do believe that the role of the physician is not going to be obsolete, at least not in our lifetimes.

So, if AI can help me to come up with an accurate diagnosis and treatment plan, I am happy to continue in my role as caregiver and partner in health. I believe that you should embrace the changes, as they are happening whether or not you adapt to or embrace them.

## *Cautionary Measures*

Just remember that AI is probably writing the essay for the applicants that you are interviewing for your practice. Be sure to ask them to type a 3-sentence sample to briefly demonstrate the skills that will be required on the job.

Ask them to write a sentence with a pen and a piece of paper in your presence. Review their essay and ask a few follow-up questions.

Call the school or last employer and look up the telephone number yourself. Call the author of the reference letter and make sure that it actually came from them. Call the school and make sure that they actually attended the institution and look the telephone number up yourself.

With all the glory of artificial intelligence and technological advancement comes all the burden. Unfortunately, you must be diligent and cautious. And even in the age of artificial intelligence, don't forget to read, study, look things up, and follow your gut.

Believe it or not, it is possible for artificial intelligence to give you the wrong answer. So, make sure you cross-reference and follow guidelines. Listen to yourself and do not make decisions blindly. Be ready to pivot as the environment in which we practice medicine changes, as it has always done.

The only thing that is constant...is change! By the time this book is published and reaches your hand, I have to accept that the state, current understanding and utilization of artificial intelligence will likely have already far exceeded my wildest imaginings.

We have no choice but to evolve and adapt to the changing scene in which we exist.

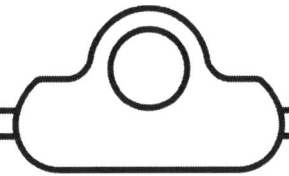

## BOTTOM LINE

Artificial Intelligence can enhance your practice.

Artificial Intelligence does not have to replace you, it can be a tool.

Artificial Intelligence is here!

# ℞ ACTION PLAN

☐ Mentally prepare for the changes that will come to the way that we practice medicine.

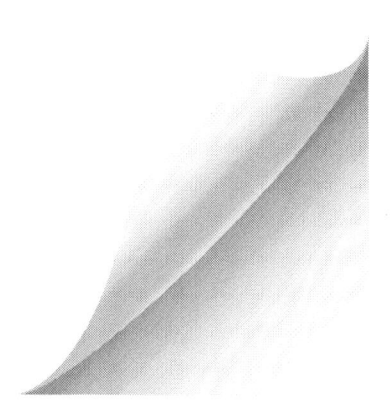

# Epilogue

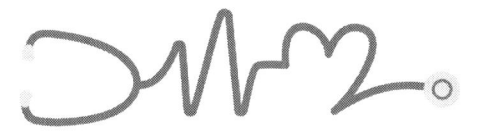

With the rapid advances in medicine and the ever-expanding wealth of knowledge that we must master, we now also have to contend with artificial intelligence and the breadth of information that patients have access to.

This can be quite potentially a very overwhelming proposal, practicing medicine that is!

Hopefully, as we have navigated some scenarios in this book, and as we have had the opportunity to see the humor in some of the things that we do each day, we will feel more empowered to be ourselves and to pour our personalities into who we are as physicians.

The art of medicine is so much more fulfilling to explore when we are not shrouded in the need to be sterile and faceless.

## *Empowerment Through Self-Discovery*

As we have journeyed 'beyond the knowledge' and uncovered the power steps on doctoring with a human touch, it is my hope that you indeed feel empowered to, despite the pressure, be yourself while being the doctor and healer that you are.

As you have mastered the factual and conceptual knowledge needed to be supremely successful on scores of exams throughout your life; may you also master deeply, through contemplating and implementing the principles explored in this work, the knowledge of yourself, your style and your preferences. May you allow yourself to display your mastery to your patients, to yourself and to the world.

## *The Power Within You*

Godspeed as you unleash the great powerful force of knowledge and compassion that you are!

Within you lies the ability to teach, to heal, to empower, to motivate, to inspire, to understand, to reach out, to listen, to accept, to open up, to counsel and to be GREAT!

# Afterword

Dr. Parker-Curling is a student and master of the meticulous, no detail easily escapes her notice. She has always been one to approach a problem and calmly engage with it until it bends to her considerable will. She is never content to allow a pressing need to remain unaddressed and, instead, would make it her business to see it resolved.

Her Beyond The Knowledge Project reflects these core elements of her personality. Having become a brilliant doctor, specialist, public speaker, teacher, wife, and mother, Dr. Parker-Curling, as one who has achieved as much as she has must do, looked back on her challenges, trials, triumphs, and the insights gained along her journey and said, "if only I had known this then!".

What for most would have been a passing, possibly recurring, lamentation, instead lit a fire in her that led to the book you have just completed, which I believe will be an important resource for medical students, physicians, healthcare providers, and patients for years to come.

Dr. Parker-Curling is driven by igniting the spark of a fresh understanding in others and by the excitement that putting knowledge into practice brings. She is determined to leave no relevant audience unreached or issue unexplored on her mission to take us all beyond our own expectations, understanding, and perceived horizons.

Ultimately, this work is an ode to the patient, whose care and wellbeing truly motivates my sister. It is my hope that the givers of care who read this book embrace its message and appreciate that it is the feeling of accomplishment that they experience when a patient says "thank you for helping me better understand my needs and options. I don't normally feel this safe, seen, and understood" that is Dr.Kristine Parker-Curling's "Why".

I am certain that she has bestowed the honour and privilege of writing this Afterword upon me in order to keep herself accountable to her mission to give of herself fearlessly, the achievement of which is reflected on every page. She can rest assured that she has successfully given you, the reader, a truly impactful, practical, and special tool to make certain you get the most out of your experiences as a medical student, physician, caregiver, or patient.

If you happen to be reading this before you embark upon an engagement with this work, I am truly excited for you, because you get to approach the experience confident and reassured of a meaningful return on the investment of your time.

I encourage you to journey with Dr. Kristine Parker-Curling, trust me, you will be in the safest pair of hands I know.

*Kahlil D. Parker KC*

# Acknowledgments

To my parents; Mr. and Mrs. Cedric and Josephine Parker, who poured so much into me and into each of my siblings, helping to shape us into who and what we are and who we continue to become.

To my father who supported us financially, sparing no cost to himself.

To my mother, my armor bearer and prayer warrior, I thank you! Your knees are not dark for nothing! You continue to bear us up in prayer, and for this, I am truly thankful.

To Kahlil, the holder of many of my secret dreams and aspirations...You know where we are going Kai.

To my brothers as a collective (Kahlil, Neil, Miles, and Quincy) who always love and support me no matter what.

To Neil my roommate, Miles our leader, and Quincy the adventurer. No one captures it quite like Rudyard Kipling does; 'For the strength of the pack is the wolf, and the strength of the wolf is the pack' (Jungle Book). I love my wolfpack. I could not have been born into a better one.

To my husband, DuVaughn, who from before we wed, has never ceased to put my needs before his own, I see you baby and, I love you endlessly.

To my children, whom I love with more love than I knew that I had, thank you for sharing your mommy with so many.

To my EJ Rolle people, we are walking in divine favor y'all.

To my best friends, my girls, thank you for always helping me to believe in myself.

To Rawi and Lenci, we are doing this!

To the Curlings, thank you for always showing up and for taking care of the kiddies tirelessly.

To my mentors (Both living and beyond), teachers, friends, and all those who contributed to shaping me into the adult human that I continue to evolve into, thank you.

To my patients, thank you for allowing me to participate in your care and to learn from you.

To my sources of inspiration and pastoral leaders, some of whom I have only interacted with virtually, I thank God for you.

To my other spiritual mentors and supporters, thank you and thank God for leading you to me.

To my God and savior, thank you for ordering my steps and directing my path.

To all the things that have led me to this point, things seen and unseen, known and unknown, I acknowledge that all of my strength comes from the Lord and that all things work together for my good!

# Bonus Resources

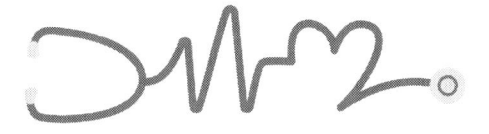

As we wrap up our journey beyond the knowledge, I want to leave you with some practical tools to help bring the C.A.R.E. framework into your daily practice.

In the following pages, you'll find a wealth of resources to support your growth as a compassionate healthcare provider.

First, you'll see a list of the 17 Power Steps we've explored throughout this book.

This serves as a quick reminder of the key concepts we've covered - from the Power of Compassion to Doctoring in the Age of AI. Keep this list handy as a roadmap for your ongoing journey in humanizing healthcare.

You'll also find a C.A.R.E. Framework Quick Reference Guide, a Self-Assessment Questionnaire, and a Self-Care Sheet.

These aren't just add-ons – they're your companions in this ongoing journey of compassionate care.

Additionally, I've included a collection of prayers that have helped me through my career. While this isn't a religious book, I'm sharing what works for me, hoping it might be a help for someone else.

Use these tools. Adapt them.

Let them remind you of the human touch that makes all the difference in our profession.

Remember, we're all works in progress, constantly learning and growing. These resources are here to support you as you continue to develop into the kind of doctor that even other doctors seek out.

So take a deep breath, flip the page, and let's put C.A.R.E. into action!

# POWER STEPS

## YOUR GUIDE TO COMPASSIONATE C.A.R.E.

Throughout this book, we've explored 17 key "Power Steps" that can transform your practice and deepen your connection with patients.

These steps are organized within our C.A.R.E. framework - Compassion, Awareness, Responsiveness, and Engagement. Each step represents a skill or mindset that can elevate your doctoring from good to exceptional.

As you review this list, reflect on which areas you excel in and which might need more attention. Remember, mastering these steps is a lifelong journey. We're all works in progress, constantly growing and improving.

Use this list as a quick reference when you need inspiration or a reminder of the many ways you can bring a human touch to your practice. Whether you're facing a challenging patient interaction or adapting to new technologies, these Power Steps will guide you towards more compassionate, effective care.

Let's review these powerful tools that can help you to become the doctor that even doctors go to for doctoring. Each step is a building block in creating a medical practice that goes beyond knowledge, helping you to truly C.A.R.E. for patients.

# POWER STEPS

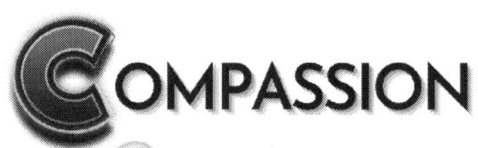

## Compassion
1. COMPASSION
2. ACKNOWLEDGMENT
3. COURTESY

## Awareness
4. PHYSICAL POSITIONING
5. LISTENING
6. EYE CONTACT

## Responsiveness
7. TOUCH
8. EFFECTIVE COMMUNICATION
9. TRUST
10. REFERRING
11. PROFESSIONALISM IN YOUR OFFICE

## Engagement
12. RELATABILITY
13. NAVIGATING DIFFICULT PATIENT SITUATIONS WELL
14. SERVING AS DOCTOR TO A DOCTOR
15. CARING FOR A PATIENT WHOSE FAMILY MEMBER IS A DOCTOR
16. DOCTORING IN THE AGE OF TELEMEDICINE
17. DOCTORING IN THE AGE OF AI

## COMPASSION

Show Genuine Concern For Patient Well-Being

Practice Empathy and Active Listening

Acknowledge Patient Emotions and Experiences

Remember Self-Compassion and Colleague Support

## AWARENESS

Be Present In Each Patient Interaction

Pay Attention To Non-Verbal Cues and Body Language

Recognize Personal Biases and Their Potential Impact

Stay Mindful Of The Patient's Cultural Background

# C.A.R.E. FRAMEWORK
## Quick Reference Guide

## RESPONSIVENESS

Adapt Communication Style To Patient Needs

Address Patient Concerns Promptly and Thoroughly

Remain Flexible In Approach To Treatment Plans

Continuously Assess and Adjust Care Strategies

## ENGAGEMENT

Involve Patients In Decision-Making Processes

Build Rapport Through Personal Connection

Encourage Questions and Open Dialogue

Commit To Ongoing Learning and Improvement

# SELF-CARE ESSENTIALS FOR PHYSICIANS

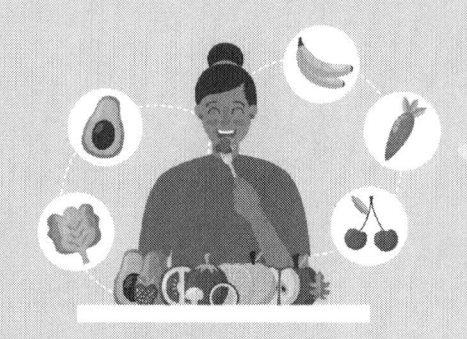

BALANCED DIET

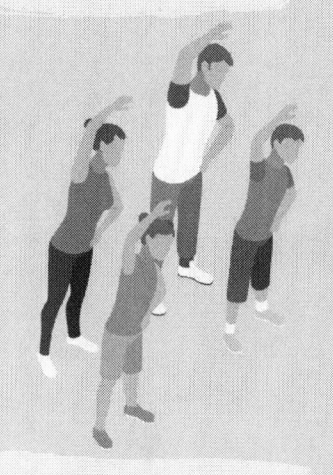

EXERCISE

REST

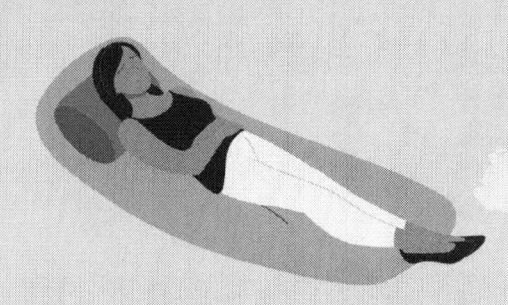

GRATITUDE

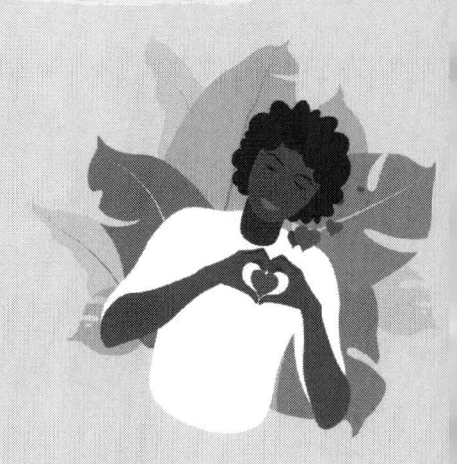

TIME MANAGEMENT

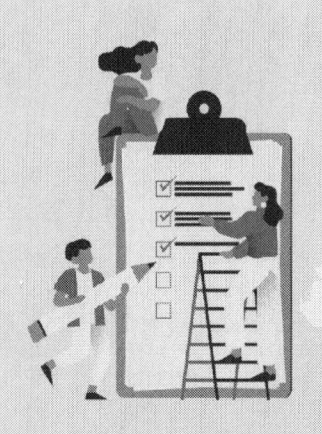

# C.A.R.E. FRAMEWORK
## SELF-ASSESSMENT QUESTIONNAIRE

### INSTRUCTIONS:
Rate yourself on a scale of 1 (needs improvement) to 5 (excellent) for each C.A.R.E. Component:

### QUESTIONS | RATING SCALE:

**RATING SCALE:** 1  2  3  4  5

### COMPASSION

- I consistently show empathy towards my patients.
- I take time to listen to my patients' concerns without interrupting.
- I acknowledge and validate my patients' emotions.
- I practice self-compassion and support my colleagues.

**TOTAL FOR COMPASSION:**

### AWARENESS

- I give my full attention to each patient during interactions.
- I notice and respond to patients' non-verbal cues.
- I'm aware of my own biases and work to minimize their impact.
- I consider cultural factors in patient care.

**TOTAL FOR AWARENESS:**

### SCORING FOR EACH COMPONENT

| | |
|---|---|
| 16-20: | Excellent |
| 11-15: | Good |
| 6-10: | Fair |
| 1-5: | Needs Improvement |

# C.A.R.E. FRAMEWORK
## SELF-ASSESSMENT QUESTIONNAIRE

### INSTRUCTIONS:
Rate yourself on a scale of 1 (needs improvement) to 5 (excellent) for each item:

| QUESTIONS | RATING SCALE: |
|---|---|
| | 1  2  3  4  5 |

### RESPONSIVENESS

- I adjust my communication style based on patient needs.
- I address patient concerns promptly and thoroughly.
- I'm flexible in adjusting treatment plans when necessary.
- I regularly reassess and modify care strategies.

**TOTAL FOR RESPONSIVENESS:**

### ENGAGEMENT

- I involve patients in their care decisions.
- I build personal connections with my patients.
- I encourage patients to ask questions and express concerns.
- I actively seek opportunities for both professional and personal growth.

**TOTAL FOR ENGAGEMENT:**

| SCORING FOR EACH COMPONENT | OVERALL TOTAL |
|---|---|
| 16-20: Excellent | 61-80: Excellent |
| 11-15: Good | 41-60: Good |
| 6-10: Fair | 21-40: Fair |
| 1-5: Needs Improvement | 1-20: Needs Improvement |

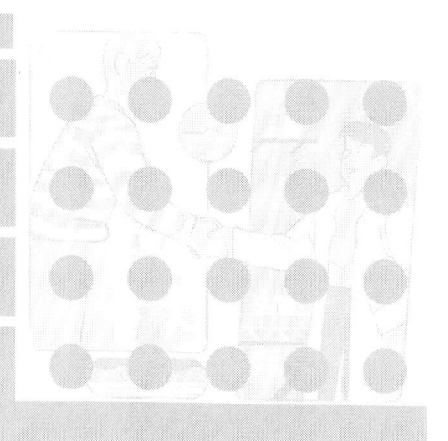

# PRAYERS FOR PHYSICIANS

## A PRAYER FOR STRENGTH

"Lord, grant me the strength to face today's challenges with compassion and grace.
Help me to see Your light in every patient I encounter.
Amen."

## A PRAYER FOR WISDOM

"Heavenly Father, guide my hands and my mind as I care for my patients.
Grant me the wisdom to make the right decisions and the humility to know when to seek help.
Amen."

## A PRAYER FOR COMPASSION FOR MYSELF

"Dear Lord, help me to remember to care for myself as I work tirelessly to care for others.
Amen."

# Endnotes

The Power of Compassion

1. Lunch, M. (2023, May 11). Graduation rates and attrition rates of U.S. medical students. *The Edvocate*. Retrieved May 16, 2023, from https://pedagogue.app/graduation-rates-and-attrition-rates-of-u-s-medical-students/

2. Lunch, M. (2023, May 11). Graduation rates and attrition rates of U.S. medical students. *The Edvocate*. Retrieved May 16, 2023, from https://pedagogue.app/graduation-rates-and-attrition-rates-of-u-s-medical-students/

3. MedEdits. (2023). Medical school acceptance rates, admissions statistics + average MCAT and GPA for every medical school (2023-2024). *Medical school average GPA & MCAT, admissions statistics and acceptance rates (2023)*. Retrieved May 16, 2023, from https://www.mededits.com

4. Proverbs 18:16, NIV

5. Proverbs 4:23, NIV

The Power of Compassion

1. Andrew, L.B. (n.d.). Physician suicide: Overview, depression in physicians, problems with treating physician depression. *Medscape*. Retrieved from https://emedicine.medscape.com/article/806779-overview

2. Luke 4:1-2, 14-15; Mark 6:30-32; Matthew 14:1-13; Luke 6:12-13; Luke 22:39-44; & Luke 5:16, NIV

3. Genesis 2:1-3, NIV

The Power of Acknowledgement

1. Pellegrini, C. A. (2017, June 1). Time-outs and their role in improving safety and quality in surgery. *Bulletin of The American College of Surgeons*. Retrieved March 7, 2023, from https://bulletin.facs.org/2017/06/time-outs-and-their-role-in-improving-safety-and-quality-in-surgery/

The Power of Listening

1. Rhoades, D. R., McFarland, K. F., Finch, W. H., & Johnson, A. O. (2001). Speaking and interruptions during primary care office visits. *Family Medicine*, 33(7), 528-532. PMID: 11456245. Retrieved March 7, 2023, from https://pubmed.ncbi.nlm.nih.gov/11456245/

The Power of Eye Contact

1. Montague, E., Chen, P., Xu, J., Chewning, B., & Barrett, B. (2013). Nonverbal interpersonal interactions in clinical encounters and patient perceptions of empathy. *Journal of Participatory Medicine*, 5.

2. Northwestern University. (2013, October 16). Eye contact builds bedside trust. *ScienceDaily*. Retrieved from https://www.sciencedaily.com/releases/2013/10/131016100447.htm

3. Kahn, A., Smith, B., & Doe, C. (2014). Patient attitudes toward physician nonverbal behaviors during consultancy: Results from a developing country. *ISRN Family Medicine*, 2014, Article ID 473654. https://doi.org/10.1155/2014/473654

The Power of Touch

1. Kahn, A., Smith, B., & Doe, C. (2014). Patient attitudes toward physician nonverbal behaviors during consultancy: Results from a developing country. *ISRN Family Medicine*, 2014, Article ID 473654. https://doi.org/10.1155/2014/473654

2. Osmun, W. E., Brown, J. B., Stewart, M., & Graham, S. (2000). Patients' attitudes to comforting touch in family practice. *Canadian Family Physician*, 46, 2411–2416.

3. Cater, A., Johnson, B., & Lee, C. (2012). Touch in the consultation. *British Journal of General Practice*, 62(569), 147-148.

4. Urick, S. (n.d.). The healing power of touch. *Prospective Doctor*. Retrieved May 2, 2024, from https://www.prospectivedoctor.com

The Power of Professionalism In Your Office

1. Dr. Nneka Unachukwu. (2022). The EntreMD Method: A Proven Roadmap for Doctors Who Want to Live Life and Practice Medicine on Their Terms. Publisher: EntreMD Publishing

The Power of Relatability

1. National Heart, Lung, and Blood Institute. (2021, December 29). DASH eating plan. *National Heart, Lung, and Blood Institute*. Retrieved April 7, 2024, from https://www.nhlbi.nih.gov/education/dash-eating-plan

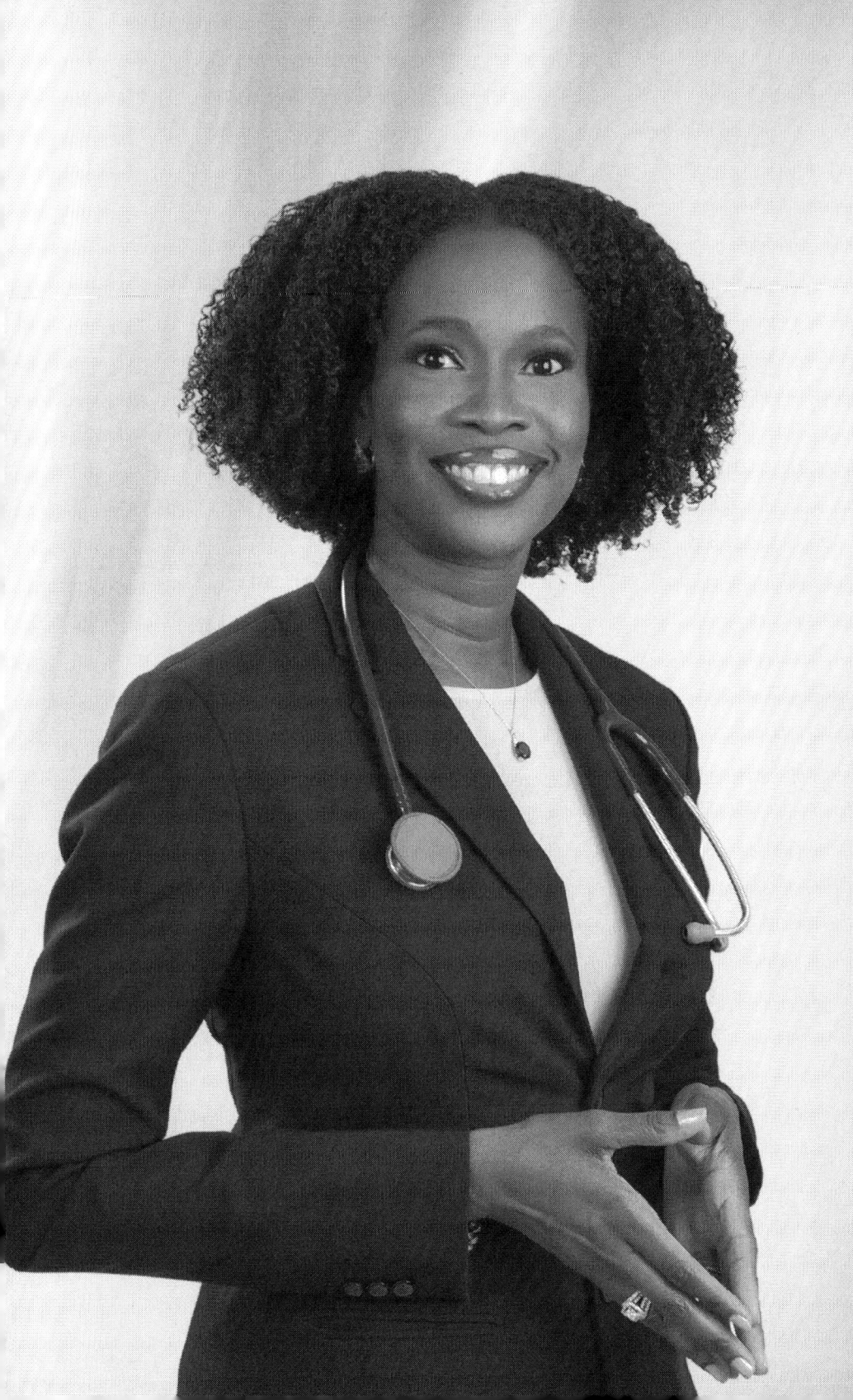

# Meet Dr. Kristine

Dr. Kristine Parker-Curling is a compassionate physician, author, and advocate for humanizing healthcare. Raised in a family that values hard work, prayer, and excellence, she carries these principles into her medical practice and writing.

After graduating from Queen's College high school in Nassau, Bahamas, her formal education began with an Associate's Degree in Biology and Chemistry from the College of The Bahamas. She then matriculated to McMaster University where she graduated Suma Cum Laude, with an Honours Degree in Biology and Psychology. Dr. Parker-Curling then pursued her medical education at The University of the West Indies in both Jamaica and The Bahamas. Her exceptional performance led to her graduating as most outstanding student (valedictorian) of her graduating class of 2007. She received her medical degree with honors.

Dr. Parker-Curling's journey continued with an Internal Medicine Residency at The State University of New York (SUNY) in Brooklyn, followed by a Fellowship in Endocrinology, Diabetes, and Metabolism at The Medical University of South Carolina, in Charlston. While practicing endocrinology in Delaware, she furthered her education, becoming specialized in the discipline of obesity medicine.

Her credentials include board certifications in Internal Medicine; Endocrinology, Diabetes, and Metabolism; as well as Obesity Medicine.

Returning to The Bahamas in 2016, Dr. Parker-Curling joined the Faculty at The University of The West Indies School of Clinical Medicine & Research, Nassau, Bahamas as an Associate Lecturer. She was excited to return to her homeland, as there was no practicing Endocrinologist residing in the country at the time.

Dr. Parker-Curling's passion for compassionate care led her to develop the C.A.R.E. framework - Compassion, Awareness, Responsiveness, and Engagement. This framework, detailed in her book "Beyond The Knowledge: Power Steps On Doctoring With A Human Touch," encapsulates her belief that effective healthcare goes beyond medical knowledge to embrace the human element of patient care.

Through her writing and practice, Dr. Parker-Curling challenges healthcare professionals to cultivate these essential qualities, creating a more empathetic and effective healthcare environment. Her work bridges the gap between clinical expertise and the art of human connection in medicine.

When not seeing patients or writing, Dr. Parker-Curling enjoys athletics, music, and spending time with her family, including her husband, Dr. DuVaughn Curling, a Hematologist and Oncologist.

Her multifaceted approach to life and medicine continues to inspire both her colleagues and patients, embodying the C.A.R.E. principles she champions.

# *INDEX*

## A

**Acknowledgment, power of**

- importance in physician-patient relationships, 55-62
- making patients feel recognized, 55-57
- personal greeting techniques, 55-56
- navigating miscommunication, 56
- building therapeutic relationships through, 56-57
- embracing authenticity in interactions, 57
- practical aspects of patient identification, 57-58
- "Time Out" procedure, 58
- humanizing patient care beyond diagnosis, 58-60

**AI (Artificial Intelligence)**

- adapting to technological advancements, 257-264
- impact on healthcare, 257-264
- adapting to technological changes, 258-259
- presence in current healthcare, 258-259
- information burden and, 259-260
- as a healthcare tool, 259-260
- maintaining human touch with, 260-262
- unspoken connections not replaceable by, 261-262

- cautionary measures when using, 262-263
- physician's role in AI era, 261-262
- cross-referencing importance, 263

**Appointments**
- waiting times, impact of, 64-67
- apologizing for lateness, 64-65
- balancing needs of patients, 66-68
- double-booking, challenges of, 64
- managing patient expectations about, 65
- patient perceptions of time value, 65

**Awareness**
- as core component of C.A.R.E. framework, 7, 11-12, 75-116
- being mindful of surroundings, 75
- conscious of patients' expressions, 75
- impact of habits, behaviors, and postures, 75
- maintaining despite exhaustion, 75-76
- physical positioning impact, 79-83
- listening importance, 85-106
- eye contact significance, 109-114

## B

**Bad news, breaking**

- avoiding definitive timelines, 201-202
- careful communication importance, 202-204
- prediabetes and diabetes diagnosis, 203-205
- reframing diagnosis as opportunity, 205

**Body language**

- awareness of, 75, 83
- connecting with patients and, 83
- reading during patient interactions, 75, 83
- telemedicine challenges with, 247-255

**Burnout**

- compassion and, 22
- emotional toll of medicine, 22-25
- prevention strategies, 43-45, 51-52

## C

**C.A.R.E. framework**

- overview and structure, 7, 11-15
- Compassion component, 7, 11, 17-54
- Awareness component, 7, 11-12, 75-116
- Responsiveness component, 7, 12-13, 117-174

- Engagement component, 7, 13-14, 175-264
- application in various settings, 12
- as acronym and teaching tool, 11

**Cancer patients**
- addressing fertility concerns, 222-223
- addressing sexual concerns, 222-224
- breaking bad news to, 201-204

**Chaperones, use of**
- for physical examinations, 127-128
- when touching patients, 128

**Clinical skills**
- clinical acumen development, 90-91
- balancing with communication skills, 90-91
- diagnostic value of listening, 93-98
- documentation importance, 90-91
- physical examinations, power of touch in, 121-128

**COVID-19 pandemic**
- impact on telemedicine, 247-248
- isolation effects, 121-122
- paradigm shift in healthcare delivery, 247

**Communication, effective**

- adapting to patient needs, 139-144
- barriers to, 131-138
- basic principles of, 131-133
- building trust through, 153-159
- cultural sensitivity in, 133-137
- in sensitive scenarios, 145-151
- non-verbal components, 109-114, 121-129
- patient education through, 179-192
- power of relatability in, 179-192
- streamlining patient encounters, 140-141
- with colleagues and staff, 169-173
- with unconscious patients, 145-149
- with physician-patients, 227-235
- with relatives of physicians, 239-245

**Compassion**

- as core component of C.A.R.E. framework, 7, 11, 17-54
- balancing with professionalism, 21-22
- challenge of vulnerability in medicine, 21-22
- coping mechanisms and, 30-31
- cultivating among colleagues, 31-41

- emotional labor of physicians, 50-52
- foundation of caregiving, 41-52
- in patient interactions, examples of, 26-28
- self-compassion importance, 41-52
- transformative power of, 26-28
- unseen struggles of healthcare professionals, 22-25

**Confidentiality**

- impact on patient trust, 153-157
- maintaining in small communities, 153-155
- navigating family relationships and, 156

**Courtesy, power of**

- apologizing when late, 64-65
- being on time, importance of, 63-65
- impact on patient satisfaction, 63-70
- mutual respect importance, 68-70

# D

**Diabetes management**

- addressing prediabetes, 203-205
- explaining hemoglobin A1C, 187-190
- patient education importance, 180-184, 185-188
- reframing diagnosis as opportunity, 205

- simplifying complex concepts, 185-186
- use of analogies for, 183-184

**Difficult patients**
- denying requests in patient's best interest, 195-198
- navigating challenging interactions, 195-200
- setting boundaries with, 197-198

**Digital health**
- telemedicine challenges, 247-255
- artificial intelligence impact, 257-264

**Documentation**
- balancing with patient interaction, 90-91
- electronic medical record challenges, 85-86
- importance in modern practice, 90-91

**Doctor as patient**
- approaching physician-patients, 227-235
- avoiding self-diagnoses from, 230-232
- cautious prescribing for, 233-234
- treating like any other patient, 227-229

**Doctor to doctor relationships**
- caring for colleagues as patients, 227-235
- consulting with peers, 162-167

- cultivating compassion among, 31-41
- family members as physicians, navigating, 239-245
- making referrals to specialists, 161-167
- mentorship importance, 35-38
- when to refer and when not to, 162-167

## E

**Electronic medical records (EMR)**
- documentation burden, 85-86, 140-141
- impact on patient interaction, 85-86
- time management with, 85-86, 140-141

**Emotional availability**
- balancing with clinical objectivity, 22
- limits of, in clinical practice, 22
- unseen struggles with, 22-25

**Empathy**
- balancing with clinical objectivity, 22-24
- communicating through touch, 121-129
- cultivating in practice, 21-31
- impact on patient satisfaction, 26-28
- in breaking bad news, 201-204
- power of acknowledgment and, 55-62

**Engagement**
- as core component of C.A.R.E. framework, 7, 13-14, 175-264
- building connections with patients, 13-14, 175-178
- navigating difficult scenarios, 195-225
- power of relatability and, 179-192
- with evolving technologies, 247-264
- with physician-patients, 227-235
- with physician family members, 239-245

**Eye contact**
- balancing with documentation needs, 109-111
- importance in communication, 109-114
- practical tips for maintaining, 112-113
- telemedicine considerations, 248-249

**F**

**Family members**
- caring for physician's relatives, 239-245
- managing expectations of, 243-244
- navigating boundaries with, 240-243
- respect for patient autonomy with, 244-245

**Fertility issues**
- addressing in cancer patients, 222-223

- cultural pressures and, 217-219
- emotional impact on patients, 218-219
- physician's own considerations, 221-222
- referring for timely intervention, 220-221
- treating patients with compassion, 220

**Financial health**
- for physicians, importance of, 234-235
- seeking professional advice for, 234-235

**H**

**Healthcare professional development**
- balancing clinical excellence with communication, 90-91
- compassion among colleagues, 31-41
- continuing education importance, 3-4
- finding balance in career, 45-49
- gaps in medical education, 4-5
- leadership and accountability, 171-172
- self-care essentials, 41-52

**HIPAA violations**
- avoiding in small communities, 153-155
- maintaining confidentiality, 153-157

## Hospital settings
- caring for physician-patients in, 233-234
- communicating with unconscious patients, 145-149
- physical positioning in, 80-81
- time management in, 86-87

## Hypertension management
- addressing medication myths, 182-183
- patient education for, 180-184
- use of analogies for, 183-184

## I

## Internship
- challenges during, 97-98
- learning from mistakes in, 97
- value of experience during, 97-98

## L

## Leadership
- accountability in healthcare, 171-172
- cultivating future leaders, 34-35
- mentorship role in, 35-38

**Listening**

- as diagnostic tool, 93-98
- beyond the obvious, 101-106
- effective communication and, 85-92
- implementing patient-centered approach, 87-89
- in telemedicine, 249
- patient interruption issues, 86
- strategies for effective, 86-90
- time management challenges, 86-87
- value of open-ended questions, 104-106

# M

**Medical errors**

- avoiding assumptions, 228-232
- preventing misdiagnosis, 101-106
- "Time Out" procedure and, 58

**Medical education**

- gaps in communication training, 4-5
- integrating essential skills into, 12
- value of internship in, 97-98

**Mental health**
- breaking stigma around, 47-49
- physician suicide risk, 47
- seeking help importance, 47-49, 224

**Mentorship**
- importance in medical training, 35-38
- standing on shoulders of, 36-38

# N

**Nonverbal communication**
- eye contact importance, 109-114
- power of touch in, 121-129
- telemedicine challenges with, 248-249

# O

**Office management**
- leadership and accountability in, 171-172
- power of professionalism in, 169-173
- staff conduct impact on retention, 171
- telephone interactions importance, 169-170

# P

**Patient autonomy**
- respecting with physician family members, 244-245

- balancing with medical recommendations, 244-245

**Patient education**
- empowerment through, 187-191
- power of analogies in, 183-184
- power of relatability in, 179-192
- simplifying complex concepts, 185-186
- storytelling effectiveness in, 189-192

**Patient-centered approach**
- implementing in practice, 87-89
- value of in chronic disease management, 87-89

**Physical examination**
- appropriate touch during, 121-129
- cultural sensitivity during, 124-126
- importance of chaperones, 127-128
- patient dignity during, 58-60

**Physical positioning**
- building rapport through, 79-83
- importance of sitting with patients, 80-81
- tailoring to clinical settings, 79-80

**Physician burnout**
- addressing personal needs, 43-45

- coping mechanisms for, 70-71
- emotional labor contributing to, 50-52
- prevention strategies, 43-45, 51-52

**Physician stereotypes**
- misconceptions about income, 44-45
- work-life balance misconceptions, 43-45

**Physician well-being**
- beyond medicine, finding meaning, 45-49
- breaking the stigma around mental health, 47-49
- caring for yourself, 41-52
- finding balance during training, 45-49
- financial health importance, 234-235
- reproductive considerations, 221-222
- self-care essentials, 41-52
- seeking help when needed, 47-49, 224

**Physician-patient relationship**
- building trust in, 153-159
- impact of waiting times on, 64-67
- maintaining boundaries in, 68-70
- power dynamics in, 68-70
- when physician is the patient, 227-235

**Prayers for Physicians**

- as resource, 271, 279

**Prognosis discussions**

- avoiding definitive timelines, 201-202
- careful communication in, 202-204

**Professionalism**

- balancing with compassion, 21-22
- in office management, 169-173
- in telephone interactions, 169-170
- maintaining privacy and, 170-171
- staff conduct impact on, 171

**R**

**RACE framework**

- as acronym for C.A.R.E., 11-15
- component overview, 11-15
- organization of power steps, 12

**Referring patients**

- appropriate circumstances for, 161-167
- knowing limitations and, 162-164
- power of, 161-167
- to colleagues, etiquette of, 165-167

INDEX 303

- when not to refer, 164-165
- when to refer, 161-163

**Relatability, power of**

- addressing medication myths through, 182-183
- connecting conditions with daily life, 184-185
- empowering patients through education, 187-191
- in patient education, 179-192
- navigating long-term relationships with, 188-189
- patient perspectives on treatment, 180-182
- storytelling effectiveness in, 189-192
- visualizing health conditions, 183-185

**Reproductive health**

- addressing fertility concerns, 217-224
- physician's own considerations, 221-222

**Responsiveness**

- as core component of C.A.R.E. framework, 7, 12-13, 117-174
- being sensitive to cues, 117
- effective communication and, 131-151
- power of trust and, 153-159
- power of touch and, 121-129
- professionalism in office, 169-173

- referring appropriately, 161-167

## S

**Self-care**

- balancing with patient care, 41-52
- emotional labor and need for, 50-52
- finding balance during training, 45-49
- importance for healthcare providers, 41-52
- mental health considerations, 47-49
- seeking help when needed, 47-49, 224

**Self-compassion**

- as foundation of caregiving, 41-52
- embracing own needs, 46-47
- foundation for patient care, 52

**Sexual concerns**

- addressing in cancer patients, 222-224
- discussing with adolescents, 210-211
- importance of discussing, 209-211
- in various medical specialties, 213-214

**Small communities, practicing in**

- confidentiality challenges in, 153-155
- practical considerations for, 154-155

## Staff management

- accountability in healthcare, 171-172
- impact on patient retention, 171
- leadership importance in, 171-172

## Storytelling

- effectiveness in patient education, 189-192
- power of analogies in, 183-184

## T

## Telemedicine

- active listening and observation in, 249
- adapting to change, 252-254
- challenges and limitations of, 248
- controlling your environment for, 251-252
- dressing appropriately for, 252
- effective connections in, 248-249
- growing trend of, 249-250
- patience with technological challenges, 250-251
- power of doctoring in age of, 247-255

## Time management

- balancing documentation with patient care, 90-91
- in hospital settings, 86-87

- listening challenges with, 86-87
- patient expectations and, 65-66
- strategies for clinical practice, 86-90

**Touch, power of**
- as therapeutic tool, 121-129
- beyond clinical examination, 122-123
- cultural sensitivity with, 124-126
- healing beyond medicine through, 122-123
- importance of chaperones for, 127-128
- in clinical examination, 123-124
- navigating boundaries with, 127-128
- professional considerations for, 126-128

**Trust, power of**
- building through communication, 153-159
- confidentiality and, 153-157
- impact on patient disclosure, 153-155
- maintaining professional integrity, 156-157

## V

**Vulnerability**
- challenge in medicine, 21-22
- compassion and, 21-22

- emotional labor of physicians, 50-52
- in patient interactions, 21-28

## W

**Waiting times**

- apologizing for, 64-65
- impact on patient satisfaction, 64-67
- patient perspective on, 65-66

**Work-life balance**

- emotional labor and, 50-52
- finding during training, 45-49
- importance for physicians, 43-45
- self-care strategies for, 41-52

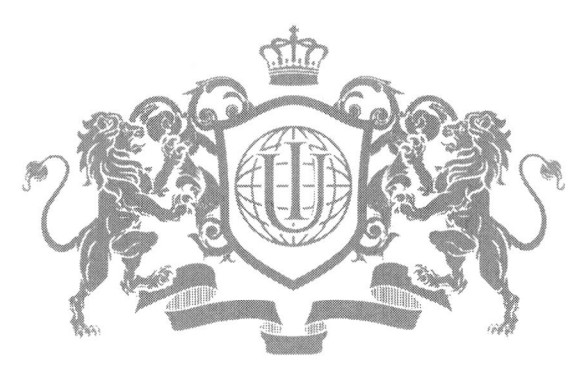

UNIVERSAL IMPACT PRESS

Made in the USA
Columbia, SC
18 April 2025